Dealing with Depre[ssion] ... of the depre-
sive illnesses, writte[n] ... ...g authorities on the
subject. The book provides a clear account of the subjective
experience, symptoms and causes of depression, as well as a
thoughtful guide to its many treatments.

Kay Redfield Jamison, PhD, Professor of Psychiatry, The Johns
Hopkins School of Medicine

Gordon Parker has written a compelling and compassionate
book about depression that makes sense, respects the intelli-
gence of the reader and is honest concerning available facts—a
rare achievement in the field.

Anthony W. Clare, MD, St Patrick's Hospital, Dublin

DEALING WITH DEPRESSION

A commonsense guide to mood disorders

BY GORDON PARKER

with the assistance of David Straton, Kay Wilhelm,
Phillip Mitchell, Marie-Paule Austin, Kerrie Eyers and
Dusan Hadzi-Pavlovic

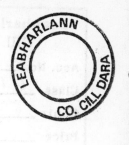

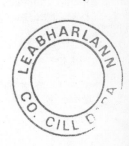

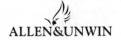

ALLEN&UNWIN

First published in 2002

Copyright © Gordon Parker 2002

Allen & Unwin
83 Alexander Street
Crows Nest NSW 2065
Australia
Phone: (61 2) 8425 0100
Fax: (61 2) 9906 2218
Email: info@allenandunwin.com.au
Web: www.allenandunwin.com

National Library of Australia
Cataloguing-in-Publication entry:

Parker, Gordon, 1942– .
  Dealing with depression: a commonsense guide to mood disorders.

  Bibliography.
  Includes index.
  ISBN 1 86508 513 8.

  1. Depression, Mental—Popular works. I. Title

616.8527

Set in 11/14 pt Sabon by DOCUPRO, Canberra
Printed by McPherson's Printing Group

10 9 8 7 6 5 4 3 2 1

People seem to be able to bear or tolerate depression as long as there is the belief that things will improve.

Kay Jamison, *Night Falls Fast*

Contents

normal depression and non-melancholic depression from
melancholic and psychotic depression, in particular, are
detailed.

of anger may feel better but those around them may feel
worse. Anger management is described.

Acknowledgments

Dealing with Depression has been written with close assistance from a number of psychiatrists associated with or working at Sydney's Prince of Wales Hospital's Mood Disorders Unit, including David Straton, Kay Wilhelm, Phillip Mitchell and Marie-Paule Austin. Its preparation was also assisted by two other Mood Disorders Unit colleagues, Dusan Hadzi-Pavlovic who gave cogent advice and Kerrie Eyers who helped at every stage with a number of demanding tasks. My secretary, Yvonne Foy, smoothed each step of the production. I am also appreciative of support from international colleagues Anthony Clare and Kay Jamison. The editorial attention provided by Allen & Unwin has been exceptional and I particularly wish to acknowledge the assistance of Rebecca Kaiser.

I am most appreciative of support from a number of leading Australian political figures who have addressed the need to increase education and training in regard to the management of depression in Australia. These include the Hon. Bob Carr, Premier of New South Wales, the Hon. Craig Knowles, the New South Wales Minister for Health, and Mr Jeff Kennett. Support for this book has also been provided by the New South Wales Department of Health, principally via the Mental Health Branch and its head, Professor Beverley Raphael.

The Mood Disorders Unit has functioned as a clinical research unit for 15 years, with its research supported by the National Health and Medical Research Council (NHMRC).

We are keen for much of its research findings and clinical wisdom to be communicated more broadly. In this, we have been assisted by the formation of the Mood Disorders Research Centre at the University of New South Wales, and by the establishment of the Black Dog Foundation—its Board (chaired by Peter Joseph OAM) comprising distinguished public and professional men and women.

There is movement at the station, for the word is getting around—depression is treatable.

Gordon Parker

List of tables and figures

☆ Tables

☆ Figures

Introduction

Depression is . . . a noun with a bland tonality and lacking
any magisterial presence, used indifferently to describe an
economic decline or a rut in the ground, a true wimp of a word
for such a major illness.

William Styron, *Darkness Visible*

Others imply that they know what it is like to be depressed
because they have gone through a divorce, lost a job or broken
up with someone. But these experiences carry with them feelings. Depression, instead, is flat, hollow and unendurable.

Kay Jamison, *An Unquiet Mind*

Depression is one of today's most common, and most commonly misdiagnosed, psychological illnesses. While I cannot
claim to cover every aspect of depression or offer any miracle
cures, *Dealing with Depression* is written for those suffering
depression themselves, the families and friends of those with
depression and professionals who want to know more about
the different treatments of depression.

In attempting to make people aware of the high incidence
of depression and its impact on the community, definitions of
'depression' have been progressively redefined and overly sim-
plified in communications to patients and to the public. The
current dominant model views depression as an 'it', that is, a
single entity rather than a set of conditions, varying only in
severity, and having nothing to do with an individual's personality (thus being beyond the individual's control). Instead,

1

depression is seen as reflecting chemical changes in the brain and therefore requiring antidepressant medication—with all antidepressant drugs being of equal effectiveness. If drugs are not favoured by either the practitioner or patient, then psychotherapy is viewed as being of comparable effectiveness and use.

Such a model is rather like viewing all skin cancers as the same and applying the same treatments to them on the basis of preference, whereas we know that there are many types of skin cancer, all triggered by different factors, some environmental, some genetic. We also know that there are many different treatments for skin cancers, each specific to the type of cancer diagnosed.

Research at the Mood Disorders Unit (MDU) in Sydney has challenged many of the current assumptions about depression. Those of us working at the unit do not view 'depression' as an 'it' but suggest that there are multiple expressions, which can represent diseases, disorders or reactions. For some depressive diseases, chemical changes in the brain may be a primary cause, with the depression occurring independently of personality and temperament; while for other depressive disorders, the individual's personality style may be all important.

We also argue against the view that the available antidepressant drugs are equally effective. We suggest that the most effective therapies are not the same for each principal depressive type, with some expressions of depression most likely to respond to antidepressant medication and others quite unlikely to respond. Similarly, we suggest that the usefulness of some of the psychotherapies (such as Cognitive Behavioural Therapy) is not equivalent across the depressive types.

In journal papers and conference presentations the Mood Disorders Unit team continues to challenge the 'dumbed down' view of depression, and believes that it is also important to communicate the challenge more widely. Such issues therefore shape the content and objectives for this book.

A diagnosis of 'depression', therefore, is only half the answer. The first question that should be asked is 'What type?'. Once the specific type of depression has been identified, patients (and their families) can be better informed about the specific causes of and treatments for the depression. Patients are thus offered a much better chance of managing, or beating, their mood disorder.

Lewis Wolpert, a Professor of Biology in London, has recently written about his episode of depression:

> I had never been seriously depressed before. I have to admit that I rather sneeringly proclaimed that I believed in the Sock School of Psychiatry—just pull them up when feeling low. But that certainly does not work with serious depression . . . It was the worst experience of my life.[1]

Wolpert wondered whether his depression had been caused by a recent social event, medication he was taking for his heart, a family tendency to depression, cultural factors or difficulties in his childhood. Readers of his book and other personal accounts might well conclude that the cause of his depression— whether genetic or environmental, biological or psychological—must therefore be the cause of other people's depressive disorders, a logical conclusion if depression is an 'it'. If depression has multiple expressions and causes—as argued here—it is wise not to assume that factors relevant to one person's depression are relevant to all.

This book provides an overview of the highs and lows of mood disorders, and of available treatments. More importantly, it describes the different principal depressive sub-types, together with their distinctive features, contributory factors or triggers and available treatments. I hope that *Dealing With Depression* will show patients and their families that there are preferential options available to them, and enable them to deal more proactively with their condition.

This is not a self-help guide, however, and I would strongly urge any significantly depressed person either to seek treatment or, at least, be assessed by a professional. Different approaches and treatments suit different people so I am not going to stipulate that you must consult *either* a general practitioner, a psychiatrist, a psychologist *or* a counsellor—everyone has access to different resources and facilities. Chapter 13 will take you through the assessment procedure and, hopefully, enable you to ask the relevant questions of your practitioner.

I will first define the various types and sub-types of depression, while demonstrating how common the condition is. The World Health Organization has estimated that over 150 million people throughout the world live with clinical depressive disorders, and that's not counting all of us who feel blue from time to time! I will then describe the principal clinical disorders, their triggers and their biology, before discussing the assessment procedures used by professionals and what to do once the diagnosis has been made.

Finally, we look at ways of beating depression. After noting the various treatments, both pharmaceutical and psychological, guidelines for matching the treatment to the illness are provided. The final chapter considers the role of family and friends, and how best to help—and cope with—someone living with depression.

1

What is depression?

> Depression is a disorder of mood . . . [which] remains nearly incomprehensible to those who have not experienced it in its extreme mode, although . . . 'the blues' . . . give many individuals a hint of the illness in its catastrophic form.
>
> William Styron, *Darkness Visible*

Depression means different things to different people. All of us, at one time or another, will have felt 'depressed', whether over bad news, a day-to-day problem, or even for no reason at all. This is described as *normal depression* or a normal *depressive mood state*. It may be experienced as a 'blue' mood, a drop in self-esteem or self-value, increased self-criticism, a lack of pleasure in life, feelings of wanting to 'give up', and pessimism about the future. Such feelings are usually not held at great depth and are transient (usually lasting only minutes to a few days).

A person suffering from *clinical depression* holds these mood state features with more conviction than someone experiencing normal depression. The mood state and associated symptoms (described on pages 6–8) will nearly always have been present for more than two weeks, and will be associated with both social and psychological disability.

Below is a representative list of features of depression, some of which indicate particular depressive disorder sub-types (these will be expanded upon in later chapters). Somebody with depression may experience:

- *Lowered self-esteem;* that is, a loss of normal self-confidence, feelings of worthlessness and inadequacy, or guilt. Pessimistic and self-critical thoughts are common.
- *Change in sleep patterns;* that is, insomnia, or broken or fitful sleep. Some people might get off to sleep at the normal time, but wake at 2–3 am and then either not get back to sleep or sleep fitfully, waking up several more times during the night. Others may take hours to get off to sleep, or sleep fitfully all night.
- *Change in mood control.* Although the word 'depression' suggests that mood is always 'down', during a depressive episode *all* moods tend to be hard to control. Some people may feel unduly miserable and pessimistic, crying for little reason and not feel any better after a good cry. Others may have difficulty controlling anger, flying off the handle at the slightest provocation. Irritability may be high, often followed by self-reproach and guilt. Anxiety can also get out of control with 'mountains being made out of mole-hills', and worrying becoming excessive. Some people develop panic attacks.
- *Change of mood through the day ('diurnal variation').* Usually people feel most depressed in the morning and improve as the day goes on, though some people experience the reverse pattern, or no mood variation at all.
- *Change in appetite and weight.* This may take two forms. In some people, especially if older, appetite may be reduced and weight lost. Constipation can also be a problem. However, for others, appetite and weight may increase. This latter pattern occurs especially in people who feel needy and respond by bingeing to cravings for sweet foods or who drink more alcohol than usual. Similarly, many people crave cigarettes when depressed.
- *Change in capacity to experience and anticipate pleasure.* Typically, hobbies and interests 'drop off'. People suffering from this symptom, termed **anhedonia**, 'just can't be bothered' to do the things that previously gave them pleasure.

- *Change in the ability to tolerate pain.* Physical pains that are normally bearable may seem to get worse, or pains may be experienced that the doctor can't explain.
- *Change in sex drive.* This is almost always reduced or absent. Occasionally, however, there is an increase in 'needy' sex, perhaps in response to depression impairing the capacity to feel close to one's partner.
- *Suicidal thoughts.* It is common to feel that there's just no point in going on. This may extend to thoughts of death, as well as to vague or specific suicidal thoughts or plans.
- *Impaired concentration and memory,* causing some people to believe they may be 'dementing' or going mad. These intellectual functions return to normal when the depression is relieved.
- *Loss of motivation* and drive. Everyday activities may seem meaningless.
- *Increase in fatigue,* feeling tired and lacking in energy. Some people may also find it hard to concentrate and may feel 'slowed down'.
- *Change in movement.* Some depressed people become physically slow or even immobile and experience slowed thinking ('retardation'). Conversely, others may become more 'agitated' and be unable to sit still, with excessive and persistent worrying causing profound mental stress. In some cases retardation may oscillate with agitation. Such obvious movement irregularity is called 'psychomotor disturbance' or PMD.
- *Psychotic features.* A small percentage of people suffering depression may develop **delusions** (false beliefs such as 'I am totally worthless', 'I am so guilty, I should be punished') and/or hallucinations (hearing voices and seeing things that are not there). Some people may note changes in their hearing and their sense of smell (often such senses are sharpened) or changes to taste.

Table 1.1   Common features of clinical depression

Reduced:	Changed from 'normal':	Varying:
• self-esteem	• appetite and weight	• mood through the day
• motivation	• sleep pattern	• emotions (such as gloom, anger, anxiety)
• sex drive		
• ability to enjoy things	*Other characteristics:*	
• pain tolerance	• movement disorder —either agitated or 'retarded', called 'psychomotor disturbance'	*Increased:*
• concentration and memory		• tiredness
		• lethargy
		• hopelessness
	• person becomes out of touch with reality —this is infrequent	• pessimism
		• apathy
		• impulsiveness
	• suicidal thoughts	• recklessness
	• impulsiveness and recklessness	

☆ False positives

So, while all of the mood state features listed above may indicate depression, most by themselves do not. For example, changes in sleep patterns can be attributed to a number of reasons. Older people generally require less sleep. Sometimes early morning waking indicates a weak bladder or a snoring partner. Being 'stressed', in itself, commonly disrupts sleep.

Changes in mood control could be the result of excessive use of alcohol or drugs or just a matter of personality style. Anxiety and panic attacks often occur separately from depression, while changes in appetite and to weight could be due to other medical conditions or as a result of medication, stress or grief.

Sex drive is liable to be reduced when there are relationship problems.

2

Depression, a common experience

Depression is referred to as 'the common cold of the psyche'. Most people will experience episodes of 'normal depression'. However, 25 per cent of women and 20 per cent of men will experience episodes of 'clinical depression' during their lifetime. Having a depressive episode is therefore commonplace and certainly no cause for shame.

What *is* a shame is that 'clinical depression' is often undiagnosed and untreated (or under-treated). This can sometimes happen because of the fear of disgrace associated with depression; or because doctors or health professionals don't recognise depression for what it is. It can also occur because individuals may not recognise their own depression. Depression may come on as a conviction that this is the way the world is or, more indirectly, physically as a series of illnesses, aches and pains.

Some clinical depressive disorders seem to run in families, with family members prone to depression, or to mood swings, in the same way other families have a tendency to stomach ulcers, diabetes or migraines. However, for many people there is no family history of depression.

If the depression is minor or transient, it may resolve by itself and not require any intervention. If it is more intrusive and persistent, professional help should be sought. When the disorder becomes intractable and debilitating, specialist treatment is required.

Those who don't respond to initial treatment may require expert review. Some people need to try several different antidepressant medications, while others need to try quite different non-medication approaches. Such varying outcomes sometimes reflect the preference of the depressed individual or treating therapist. At other times, the outcomes reflect the nature of the differing depressive disorder and the fact that the ideal or best treatment is still not known. Sometimes, a poor outcome reflects a generally appropriate antidepressant treatment being given to the wrong depressive condition (for example, a non-melancholic disorder being misdiagnosed as melancholia and being so treated) or even to a non-depressive disorder (for example, an anxiety disorder). *This underlines the importance of ensuring that the depressive sub-type is identified.*

Remember that depression can be biological in its origin, but psychological in experience. Those suffering from depression may have to push themselves or be encouraged by someone else to seek advice or treatment. They may feel that nothing much can be done about the way they feel but, in fact, most depressive disorders can readily be cleared up.

☆ The purpose of 'normal depression'

For most people, depression (even the commonly occurring 'normal' depression) is an unpleasant experience that often interferes with day-to-day functioning.

What then is the purpose of such a painful experience? This question can be linked to another one: what is the purpose of pain? Pain has one distinct advantage—the unpleasant side effects of pain mean that most of us will go to considerable length to avoid it. For example, if we did not find heat painful, we might get too close to a fire and suffer the consequences. It is for such reasons that many nerves in our bodies have heat receptors.

In a similar way, it could be argued that 'normal' depression can be an automatic defence response or a response cued by certain situations. Such a proposition has been explored recently by the American psychiatrist Randolph Nesse[1] whose thesis is considered below, in particular how 'normal' depression may have offered a selective advantage to civilisation over time. To the extent that any of Nesse's interpretations have validity, they allow the individual to question the meaning of a 'depressed mood'.

☆ What is normal depression trying to say?

Is 'normal' depression a plea or cry for help?

It is unlikely that normal depression is a cry for help. If it is, then it is not a very useful or effective signal, as it is more likely to evoke negative responses from others.

Does depression help to conserve resources?

If someone is lethargic, has no appetite, lacks motivation and has no interest in conversation, might not such a state resemble hibernation in the animal world and be a way of conserving energy?

Nesse argues that depression is 'poorly designed' for such a purpose—at least in humans. The argument might hold for animals, where an animal continues to forage for as long as there is an adequate food source. But, when the food source runs low and the animal has to use up more energy foraging than would be obtained from eating the food, it would be wiser for the animal to stand still—even if starving—and wait for some other food source to turn up. It would stretch credibility to suggest that depression has such an advantage for humans.

Can depression resolve competition with a dominant figure?

Is depression a signal to a more 'powerful' competitor that a threat no longer exists (thus ending the conflict and the depression)? Does it represent a true wish on the part of an individual to resolve a conflict and obtain reconciliation, or is depression designed to lull the competitor into a false sense of security? Again, while of clear relevance to animals, its pertinence to humans can be questioned.

Can depression help us be more realistic in goal setting?

If a particular goal (for example, a new partner, or a new job) is starting to look 'mission impossible', somebody in a depressed mood state may feel compelled to reassess the situation before disengaging from the pursuit or escaping from the particular situation. To persist with a goal that looks unattainable requires considerable increase of effort from the normal, everyday pace of life and, if the goal is not achieved, the resultant depression will be even greater.

The argument is, then, that a depressed mood drives people away from tasks that will be unprofitable, or a waste of effort or dangerous. Failure to reach, or to renounce, a goal may be depressing in the short term, but the negative 'cost' or pain may be less than the costs and pain of persevering with the task. If a setback occurs in the pursuit of a major goal, it would make sense not to rush into chasing another significant goal. In such instances, moving into a depressive state (with symptoms such as pessimism and lack of initiative) might, as Nesse notes, 'prevent calamity even while it perpetuates misery'.

☆ Conclusions

There are several limitations to the interpretations considered by Nesse. First, they appear more relevant to animals than humans. Second, their benefits in contemporary society are not obvious. Even if true, such theorising is likely to have relevance only to 'normal depression' and perhaps to some forms of non-melancholic depression.

The answer is perhaps best addressed at the individual level. Consideration of their own patterns of behaviour might prove more useful to a depressed person, especially when the episode is over. Questions that could be asked include: 'In what circumstances do I find myself getting depressed? What then is the message? Do I want to do anything about it?'

In both 'normal' and 'non-melancholic' depression some elements of the disorder may have homeostatic capacities, assisting a return to 'normal'. Thus, sleeping excessively (as many depressed individuals do) may be an adaptive behaviour by restoring slow-wave sleep during times of stress. Carbo-hydrate cravings and eating chocolates, in particular, have comforting effects that trigger the release of endorphins to create a 'feel good' state. Eating more of certain foods may lead to an increase in the amine L-tryptophan, thus increasing the activity of serotonergic neurotransmitters in the brain, which may be disrupted during depression (see page 65–6). Just as a pregnant woman may develop an aversion to ciga-rettes and alcohol because of potential damage to the foetus, some people may lose pleasure in drinking alcohol during their depression. And while some people may no longer be interested in smoking, others develop a craving for tobacco (which might then increase the level of brain neurotransmitter, dopamine, occuring in decreased levels in some depressive disorders). Thus, some symptoms in the less 'biological' types of depres-sion may be a response to 'painful' psychological and social life situations; others may be adaptive attempts at normalising disturbed biological changes.

For the more 'biological' types of depression, such as melancholia, it is difficult to believe that such disorders are primarily adaptive or functional responses. The British satirist and writer Spike Milligan has observed: 'I cannot reassure myself that it has been worthwhile . . . I do not hold with this romantic view of depression, that it has some purpose . . . As far as I am concerned it is without a redeeming feature.'[2]

By contrast, the psychiatrist Kay Jamison has stated that, if given the choice as to whether or not she would have manic-depressive illness, she would change nothing. If she had not had the disorder, she would not have 'felt more things, more deeply; had more experiences, more intensely . . . laughed more often for having cried more often; appreciated more the springs, for all the winters . . . Even when I have been most psychotic—delusional, hallucinated, frenzied—I have been aware of finding new corners in my mind and heart'.[3]

As with winter, biological depressions exist, and test people to and beyond our comprehension of what is endurable. However, they can also provide a frame of reference for a new mood or a new season.

3

Depression classification

The history of classification of diseases in medicine is like the history of maps and charts. In the sixteenth century, early map makers in Europe asked ministers of the Church to climb their bell towers and write down everything they could see. Maps were drawn from such recordings.

The development of the magnetic compass allowed more directional accuracy, and made coastal navigation easier. Bearings could be taken from features, and the position of ships calculated. The invention of the sextant permitted the measurement of latitude; that is, distance from the Equator. This was enough to allow Christopher Columbus to cross the Atlantic safely and return home again.

But without the ability to measure longitude, whole areas of charts were left void and marked with the words, 'There be Monsters here!' The discovery of how to measure longitude was the major scientific breakthrough of the eighteenth century.

In psychiatry, early attempts at classification were a bit like the ministers climbing their bell towers: all they could do was see their patients, and write down what they saw. And while most of medicine was able to progress through the 'coastal navigation' stage, psychiatry had a more difficult task.

In much of medicine, firm objective findings clearly demarcate one disease from another. These findings can be measured—such as a blood test that confirms diabetes, a biopsy that shows a particular type of cancer, or a post-mortem that shows a clot in a coronary artery.

Psychiatric classification has had to operate, as it were, out of sight of land. There are no sharp-edged rocks or islands from which to take a bearing. So, despite the many efforts to identify specific causes of mental illnesses such as **schizophrenia**, none has been found. Even post-mortem findings, which resolve most diagnostic disputes in medicine, fail to help much in psychiatry.

As a result, maps of psychiatric disorders have been a bit vague, just as charts were before longitude could be measured. But that is changing now, and modern statistics and computer-driven research are providing better ways of knowing where in the sea of psychological phenomena we are at a particular time.

☆ The importance of depression sub-types

Does it matter that there are different depressive sub-types? This is a commonly asked question, and the answer has to be Yes. Just as an accurate position is necessary if you are going to drill for oil in the seabed, or find a good spot for fishing, so too is it very important to know that there are different types of depression.

A pigmented spot of skin may be a freckle or it may be a melanoma. Swollen ankles can reflect either heart failure or a kidney problem. Before doctors could tell the difference, successful diagnosis and therefore treatment was often due to chance.

Such is the risk of viewing depression as a single disorder, and why it is important that the principal sub-types be recognised. Depression used to be thought of as one condition, varying only in severity. Regrettably, many experts and classificatory systems still hold this view. It resembles the markings on the charts before longitude was discovered: 'There be Misery here.' Descriptive, but not specific!

The psychiatric classifications of depression that have remained beached in those shoals have provided unhelpful 'maps' of depression. Particularly confusing has been the long-standing tendency to classify depression on the basis of severity, descending from 'severe' to 'moderate' to 'mild' and, more recently, as 'sub-clinical' and 'sub-threshold'. This has held back understanding and treatment. For example, in medicine swollen ankles can be 'severe', 'moderate' or 'mild' but these descriptions will not be as important as identifying whether the swelling is due to heart problems or kidney problems. Such is the case in understanding depression.

It is very important to concede that there are different types of depression, as treatments for each type vary in relevance and usefulness—antidepressant medication might be better than psychotherapy for one type of depression, while the converse may hold for another depressive type.

It is also important to concede that while social, psychological, biological and medical conditions can all influence the nature of depression, they do not necessarily provide 'the explanation'. Even though family tendency to depression, difficulties in childhood, changing cultural trends, and even evolutionary explanations should be considered, such factors are of quite varying relevance to differing depressive 'types'. Thus, for some people, genetic factors may be the principal 'cause' and life stressors of minor relevance; for others, the reverse may hold. And, to have experienced some traumatic event does not, necessarily, make it a 'cause' of depression.

There is a famous saying that 'the beating of tom-toms will always restore the sun after an eclipse'. This reminds us that if two events occur together, we risk concluding that one must have caused the other. Thus, depression might occur for the first time in a menopausal woman—but the menopause may not itself be *the* cause. Depression may well seem a very logical outcome for someone who has experienced a long sequence of high-level stressors in their life (for example, poor parenting, childhood sexual abuse, the break-up of a marriage and a severe medical illness). While such events may seem a total explanation of the depression, they may have contributed to it only partially or have no relevance at all. The 'causes' of depression may therefore be difficult to clarify for a range of reasons. Ideally, professional assessment should clarify the relevance of possible causes and provide an accurate sub-typing diagnosis.

4

'Clinical' depression

Most people experience normal depressed moods. Such moods are usually not of major intensity, last less than two weeks, and don't interfere with ability to function. The distinction between a normal depressed mood and a depressive disorder is crucial to understanding depression.

☆ Depressive disorders

Depressive disorders are more severe than a depressed mood state, last for at least two weeks and affect functioning at home and/or work.

There are three classes of clinical depressive disorders:

- non-melancholic depression;
- melancholic depression; and
- psychotic melancholia.

Melancholic depression and psychotic melancholia are less common depressive illnesses, affecting 1–2 per cent of Western populations, with the numbers being roughly equal for men and women.

Non-melancholic depression

In comparison with the two other depressive classes, non-melancholic depression lacks specific defining features such as psychomotor disturbance (PMD), which assists in defining melancholic depression, or psychotic features, which, together with PMD, assist in defining psychotic depression. Thus, people with non-melancholic depression can usually be cheered up to some degree and are less likely to report significant concentration and memory problems. As with the other depressive disorders, those with a non-melancholic depression have a mood disorder (feel depressed, have a drop in self-esteem, and are self-critical) and experience many of the associated symptoms (such as appetite and sleep disturbance) noted in Chapter 1.

Non-melancholic depression is the most 'common' depressive disorder, affecting one in four women and one in six men in the Western world over their lifetime. It has a high '**spontaneous remission**' rate, making accurate assessments of specific treatments difficult. In fact, response rates to quite different treatment approaches (for example, antidepressant drugs, psychotherapy and counselling) are very similar.

Melancholic depression

The depressed mood state in melancholic depression is generally more severe than in non-melancholic depression and PMD is evident. This sub-type has a low spontaneous remission rate and, before effective treatments were available, could last from months to decades. Its response rate to physical treatments (for example, antidepressant drugs) is high, but minimal to non-physical treatments such as counselling or psychotherapy.

Psychotic melancholia

The depressed mood state and PMD are even more severe in psychotic melancholia than in melancholic depression, and a feature unique to this disorder is present—psychotic phenomena (delusions and hallucinations). This condition has a very low spontaneous remission rate. It responds only to physical treatments.

☆ The principal depression 'patterns'

The common patterns experienced by those with the major depressive classes are described below, together with the common patterns of 'normal' depression.

Normal mood swings

Figure 4.1   Normal mood swings

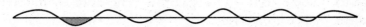

Most people experience a pattern of fairly regular 'ups and downs' (for example, being 'the life of the party' one night and glum and flat the next). Such a pattern is known as a 'cyclothymic' personality style. These swings are not severe and do not seem distinctly 'abnormal' to others.

If depression is defined as being blue, sad, hopeless and helpless, and having feelings such as wanting to give up and being pessimistic about the future, then more than 90 per cent of people will admit to such a state several times a year. While these states may range from mild to troublesome and last from minutes to hours to a couple of days, most people expect them to settle by themselves or with the use of personal coping strategies. Normal mood swings do not affect day to day functioning.

Non-melancholic depression

Figure 4.2   Mood disturbance in non-melancholic depression

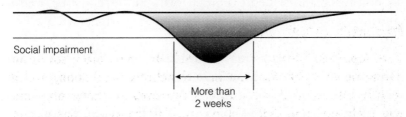

Social impairment

More than
2 weeks

In non-melancholic depression, a depressed mood is present for more than two weeks and is accompanied by social impairment (for example, difficulty in dealing with work or relationships). There is no observable PMD, nor are there psychotic features, and the features of the clinical mood state (as listed in Chapter 1) can vary. Spontaneous remission (that is, getting better naturally or 'out of the blue') is common.

There are several differing sub-types of non-melancholic depression, which are more likely to occur in people with certain personality styles (detailed on page 46) or who have a **primary** anxiety disorder (see page 50). These personality styles and the higher level of anxiety increase the risk of developing depression (and the likelihood of it persisting) when a person is faced with certain stressful events. Personality style accounts for the variable mood state features found in non-melancholic depression, and indicates why quite contrasting therapies (for example, those addressing predisposing factors, others directed at anxiety, and still others focusing on the depression) may all be quite effective.

Melancholic depression

Figure 4.3   Mood and melancholic depression

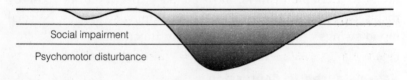

The mood state in melancholic depression is more severe than in non-melancholic depression. It lasts more than two weeks and involves moderate to severe social impairment, as well as visible PMD (for example, retardation or agitation).

Melancholic depression is primarily biological, and spontaneous remission is unusual. It tends to run in families. The first few depressive episodes may develop in response to stress, but later episodes may appear 'out of the blue' or come on after a minor problem.

Melancholic depression may also develop as a result of

exposure to certain drugs (licit or illicit) and some diseases. These can act like external stress, disrupting some of the brain's neural circuits (the basal ganglia and frontal cortex links), causing depression, PMD and concentration problems. A similar disruption happens in Parkinson's disease.

For some people, especially those without any family history of melancholia, an episode of melancholic depression can come on for the first time late in life, as age changes in the brain disrupt relevant brain (or neural) circuits. Before effective treatments became available, depression could remain for years without any relief, or before spontaneous recovery.

As noted, active physical treatments are almost invariably needed, but (as detailed later) differing antidepressant drugs range widely in their effectiveness in treating this sub-type.

Electroconvulsive Therapy (ECT) may be effective but it is rarely needed. Psychotherapy and counselling may also be used in addition to such physical treatments. However, as the main underpinning mechanism in melancholic depression is biological, not psychological, these treatments are not appropriate as primary therapies.

Psychotic melancholia

Figure 4.4   Clinical features in psychotic melancholia

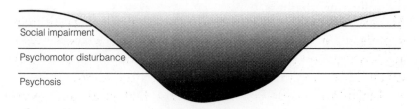

In psychotic melancholia, the depressed mood is extremely severe and present for more than two weeks. There is severe social impairment and PMD, and psychotic features (such as delusions) are evident due to additional neural circuits in the brain being disrupted. As with melancholic depression, psychotic melancholia can first appear late in life.

Preferred treatments are biological and physical, with the older antidepressant classes appearing to be more effective than many of the newer classes (see Chapter 14). However, antidepressant drugs alone are usually less effective than combination antidepressant and tranquilliser treatments (**antipsychotic** or **neuroleptic** medication), or even ECT in some instances.

☆ A 'map' of the main depressive conditions

Figure 4.5 shows the principal expressions of depressive disorders and the features that demarcate one sub-type from another. The suggestion that psychotic depression is more 'weighty' or severe than melancholic which, in turn, is more severe than non-melancholic depression is generally true. However, sub-type distinctions are driven more by the presence or absence of certain key features than by depression severity.

Most current classifications of 'depression' make distinctions on the basis of varying levels of severity. The Mood Disorders Unit argues that separate depressive classes exist, with class distinctions reflecting different causes leading to differing clinical features requiring differing treatments. The clinical disorders mapped in Figure 4.5 will be fleshed out in the following chapters.

Figure 4.5   The four principal expressions of depression and their component features

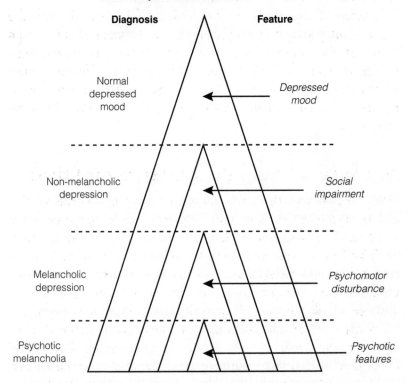

1. A *'normal' depressed mood*, not of major intensity, lasting less than two weeks, and not interfering with social functioning.
2. *Non-melancholic depression.* Depressed mood, with mood state features listed on pages 21–22, lasting more than two weeks and affecting functioning at home and/or work. No psychomotor disturbance (PMD) and no psychotic features.
3. *Melancholic depression.* The depressed mood state is generally more severe than in non-melancholic depression—and PMD is evident. No psychotic features.
4. *Psychotic melancholia.* The depressed mood state is even more (observably) severe, PMD is often very severe, and there are also psychotic features such as delusions and hallucinations.

5

Unipolar and bipolar disorders

Over time, people can exhibit quite varying patterns of mood swings. Within the clinical depressive disorders, it is important to make a distinction between unipolar and bipolar depression. The terms 'unipolar depression' or 'unipolar disorder' are used to describe a pattern of episodes of clinical depression in which there are no 'highs'. By contrast, the term 'bipolar disorder' is used to describe patterns of manic behaviour that may or may not alternate with episodes of clinical depression. Approximately 5 per cent of those suffering a bipolar disorder experience only highs. The great majority of people with the disorder alternate between highs and lows and, commonly, experience intervals of quite normal mood states in between episodes. For each individual the pattern is quite distinct. Some people with bipolar disorder might have only one episode every decade, while others may have daily mood swings.

In the past, people with severe bipolar disorder may have been admitted to an asylum where they could have remained manic for many months or depressed for many years and then spontaneously remitted, indicating that there is a pattern to even the most severe expressions of the condition. It is important to note that such severe patterns are rare. Mild bipolar patterns are common and often go undiagnosed because they may be viewed as 'normal mood swings'.

The terms 'unipolar' and 'bipolar' originally referred to the melancholic depressive sub-type but have, in the last twenty years, been broadened to refer to all expressions of clinical depression. For a clinician to tell a patient that they have a 'unipolar depression' means little more than that they have a non-bipolar disorder.

Figure 5.1   Mood swings and common clinical states in bipolar disorder

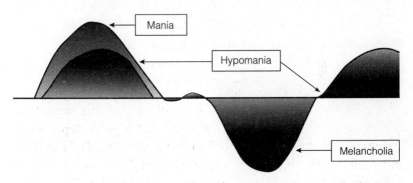

Bipolar disorder was previously called 'manic-depression' due to the swings between high and low moods. Mania is indicated by very 'high' mood (which may be expansive and/or irritable), by marked social impairment and, often, by psychotic features such as delusions and hallucinations. In hypomania, mood is still 'high', but often little more than being distinctly happy, jovial or expansive. For many, the changed mood state is obvious to others but, perhaps for the majority, the mood swing is not so marked that others would be aware of it. This explains why it is difficult to diagnose mild expressions of bipolar disorder. In some cases, the mood variation may appear to be no more than an ongoing personality style.

Bipolar disorder is biologically mediated and strongly inherited. When people develop bipolar depression, they nearly always have psychotic or non-psychotic 'melancholic' depressive episodes. There are exceptions, however. For instance, an individual with bipolar disorder may have a sequence of melancholic depressive episodes and then, when faced with an unusual stressful event (such as a job loss), develop a 'normal' depressed mood, a non-melancholic depressive disorder or a grief state.

The diagnosis of 'bipolar disorder' is not always straight-forward for several reasons, explaining why several studies have identified an average period of over ten years between the onset of the disorder and the correct diagnosis being made.

First, mild expressions can be very difficult to distinguish from a normal volatile or **cyclothymic** personality style. There are many people who swing from being 'the life of the party' to being quiet, uncommunicative and even grumpy as part of their personality style and not because they have a bipolar disorder. Creative people can experience self-induced 'highs' when caught up by the Muse: a writer, for example, may describe feeling 'taken over' during a burst of creative plan-ning, or writing in a state of excitement, needing only a few hours sleep. Some drugs will induce a sense of 'being high', both legal and illicit. Nearly all antidepressant drugs can effectively 'send' a person into a hypomanic or manic state—whether or not that individual had previously experienced a 'high' or had a tendency to do so.

Second, bipolar disorder does not always present in a classic pattern (for example, distinct highs followed by lows, or vice versa). It may commence with a period of insomnia, or follow the unexpected appearance of a physical condition such as an eating disorder, with clear bipolar depression remaining latent for months or even years.

Third, mild experiences of bipolar depression are common—particularly ones where only the individual is aware of their differing 'state', while others, even family members, may fail to detect any change.

How, then, can bipolar disorder be diagnosed with any confidence? At the Mood Disorders Unit, we explore a number of parameters with open-ended questions designed to establish whether, during any particular period, an individual has:

- experienced an elevated, euphoric, irritable or more confident mood;
- experienced reduced sleep, but without feeling tired the next day;
- had more energy or felt 'wired';
- spent more money than usual or wished to do so;
- made frivolous or unnecessary purchases;
- talked more and made more phone calls than usual;
- experienced increased libido;
- dressed more colourfully;
- been more verbally or behaviourally indiscreet than usual;
- found 'nature' more beautiful;
- been more creative;
- sung more.

It is important to understand that such features are noted relatively consistently across different cultures, although cultural factors influence their actual expression. The psychiatrist Kay Jamison documents a saying used by the Old Order Amish that suggests bipolar depression—'racing one's horse and carriage too hard'.

If there is still doubt about the diagnosis after working through the list, then it is a good idea to talk to a family member who may provide similar or even quite different information. It is also valuable to pursue the family history to determine whether any family members have had bipolar disorder (even obtaining old hospital and medical records) and to ask to see the individual when the next 'high' is experienced.

Even after pursuing all diagnostic options, for a percentage of individuals the diagnosis will remain in doubt. Their situation should generally be reviewed after an interval or, less commonly, mood stabilisers could be trialled to determine if there is any impact on their mood state and functioning.

Regrettably, the diagnosis of bipolar disorder is commonly missed for several reasons. First, some health practitioners are unaware of it or are untrained in its assessment. Second, many practitioners fail to consider it when undertaking patient assessment. Third, many patients with mild bipolar disorder enjoy their 'highs' and prefer not to tell anybody about them.

6

General features of depression and bipolar disorders: the experience

Depression can be experienced in many different ways, reflecting the individual's personality, coping repertoires and mood state, as well as the type of depression. As there are no absolute rules, definitions of 'the experience' can only be imprecise markers of depressive sub-types.

For someone experiencing depression, their general mood state will be negative and marked by pessimism, lowered self-confidence, and a sense of helplessness and hopelessness. They may want to 'walk away from things' (for example, leave a difficult job or marriage), thus risking a drop in the social hierarchy. These features are generally more severe and pervasive in melancholic and psychotic depression. By contrast, in 'normal' and 'non-melancholic' depression, individuals may be able to 'bounce out' of the mood state, perhaps in response to support from others, or to something pleasant occurring in their life.

Some people may detect certain 'gains' from experiencing depression. For example, somebody who has constantly 'won' in life and who has taken things for granted may, for the first time, appreciate others and re-evaluate life's basic priorities. It has been argued that, in such instances, the 'rosy glow' that non-depressed people can adopt to handle life's difficulties may be lost, thus ensuring issues are seen in a more objective way.

☆ Coping repertoires in 'normal' and non-melancholic depression

It is interesting to consider the coping repertoires used in dealing with or trying to overcome the depression. For example, normal or non-melancholic depression may make some people feel 'cold', and they might need to warm themselves up, perhaps by sitting in a warm bath or by sitting next to a window taking in the sun on a winter's day.

Some people may engage in self-consolatory behaviours, such as going shopping or 'pigging out' on certain foods, such as chocolate. Such behaviour can reflect complex psychological processes—'He no longer cares for me. I will therefore care for myself. I will eat something I can really enjoy'.

Others may become reckless and impulsive, and perhaps throw or smash things or drive dangerously. While recklessness is more likely in men, women may also show such behavioural patterns, perhaps through socialising or relating to men in 'at-risk' ways.

Some women may become careless and 'forget' about contraception, particularly after a break-up in a relationship. Reasons for doing so may include an attempt to re-start the relationship, or to 'keep part of him'.

A more common behaviour is to seek 're-attachment'. Many people seek help from friends and professionals, or in less direct ways such as praying. Some seek to distract themselves from the depressive thoughts either by working harder or more repetitively, or by developing a 'depressive habit' such as painting the kitchen during each episode. Others will actively seek passivity and attempt to block things out by drinking to excess, taking anxiety-relieving or sleeping tablets, or just going to bed 'to escape'. Suicidal thoughts and actions may occur even in non-melancholic disorders, but are more likely to be countered by notions such as 'I wouldn't want to hurt my children'.

Those who have an 'internalising' personality style (see pages 47–9) may retreat to their room to brood and ruminate about their hurt. They may believe themselves to be more inadequate than they actually are, ignoring their usual strengths.

Those with an 'externalising' style (see page 49) may be irritable and angry with those around them and start yelling and throwing or smashing things such as dinner sets or glassware.

Thus, in 'normal' or 'non-melancholic' depression, we see people using their inherent coping repertoires and revealing aspects of their personality as they try to cope with their mood state.

☆ Coping repertoires in melancholic depression

The mood state in melancholic depression is more dominant than in non-melancholic depression. The individual's personality style is less evident and may be 'trumped' by the mood-dominated picture. The mood state is both more severe and certainly more pervasive (there is nothing to look forward to, there is no pleasure to be found in the usual pleasurable events, interest cannot be maintained in activities) and will be present throughout the day, although it may be particularly severe in the morning. Concentration and memory function are commonly impaired. There is also an increased risk of suicide.

Observable PMD means that somebody suffering from melancholic depression can appear either 'retarded' or 'agitated', or even alternate between each state. Agitation may increase the suicide risk, while severe retardation may reduce the risk. Unfortunately, as treatment progresses and retardation decreases, those suffering melancholic depression can be at greater risk of suicide even though by all appearances they are recovering.

In 'retarded' melancholic depression, actions slow down—those suffering from this disorder may walk or talk slowly, pause before moving or talking, use briefer sentences with reduced conversational richness, and are not able to brighten (at all, superficially or temporarily) at the introduction of pleasant topics. The normal 'light in the eyes' is diminished or lost, facial movements are less mobile, hair may become brittle and skin pale and even pasty.

The novelist William Styron, in *Darkness Visible*, captures the elements of this mood state: '. . . my speech, emulating my way of walking, had slowed to the vocal equivalent of a shuffle . . . I'd feel the horror, like some poisonous fogbank, roll in upon my mind, forcing me into bed. There I would lie for as long as six hours, stuporous and virtually paralyzed'.[1]

A description of Spike Milligan, while he was experiencing an episode, also captures aspects of retardation: 'He is markedly lacking in spontaneity, sitting quietly, responding to questions but initiating little conversation. There is a noticeable lack of facial expression and little extraneous movement.'[2] And Milligan's own description: '. . . this vital spark has stopped burning . . . I go to dinner . . . and don't say a word, just sit like a dodo. It must be a bit unbalanced at the table with me sitting there dead-silent . . . It is like a light switch. I feel suddenly turned off. There is a tiredness, a feeling of complete lethargy'.[3]

Those suffering 'agitated' melancholic depression appear preoccupied with what are usually quite mundane things—which are blown out of proportion—and show considerable 'mental anxiety'. They may pace up and down, wringing their hands, or even make little picking movements. Speech is rapid but superficial, and without the usual richness—again dominated by mundane concerns. Sufferers may look apprehensive or even fearful, and their mental anguish is often visible to others.

In *An Unquiet Mind,* Kay Jamison describes one experience of agitation: '. . . I became exceedingly restless, angry, and irritable, and the only way I could dilute the agitation was to run along the beach or pace back and forth across my room like a polar bear at the zoo.'[4]

Such stereotypical presentations (of observable retardation and agitation) are usually independent of the individual's personality, and suggest to the professional observer a biological disruption or disease process. In younger people, psychomotor disturbance may be less evident. On questioning, however, they will usually describe experiencing motor changes and, in particular, effects on thinking and concentration, perhaps finding it quite impossible to study or to concentrate on reading.

The simple term 'depression' has been rejected by a number of writers as it is not capable of capturing the import of melancholic depression. William Styron suggested the term 'brainstorm' to describe 'a veritable howling tempest in the brain'.[5] The broadcaster Helen Razor felt bombarded by a 'broken head' and felt 'plagued . . . by the suspicion that my synapses were exploding . . . of phrenic crashing . . . I became immobilised by these potent little shocks . . . I would imagine that my poor battered lobes were rolling about yolklike in my feckless eggshell head'. [6]

☆ Coping repertoires in psychotic melancholia

In psychotic melancholia, the depressed mood is either extremely severe or, at times, even denied. Where depression is denied, the individual may instead describe states of nothingness, of profound enervation, or even of the disturbance being felt at the physical level (with flu-like symptoms, physical agitation or pain). Such a mood state persists across and over the days, and lacks the late in the day lift experienced by many with melancholic depression.

PMD (whether retardation or agitation) is even more severe in psychotic melancholia than in melancholia, so that in the 'retarded' state the individual's appearance may resemble that of someone with dementia. Concentration, attention and memory are generally impaired.

In agitated psychotic depression, the individual is rarely still except when asleep. A common speech pattern is that of repeated questions; for example, 'What is going to become of me?'.

Delusions are far more common than hallucinations (unless the individual has profound PMD), and many people suffer from 'mood-congruent' themes (for example, 'I am so worthless that I deserve to be put in jail or punished in some other way.'). Minor indiscretions of the past may serve as a focus for such delusional thinking and are generally blown out of proportion. Thus, someone who did not disclose two dollars on their tax return twenty years before may genuinely believe that they will be jailed for this minor indiscretion.

A percentage of people with psychotic melancholia will experience 'mood-incongruent' delusions (for example, that their home is being gassed, or that their food is being poisoned). Some delusions effectively 'build in' physical features that emerge during the episode. For example, psychotic melancholic people with constipation may believe that their bowels have turned to cement or that they have a bowel cancer. Many with psychotic melancholia have 'over-valued ideas' that are just short of being delusional, usually associated with pre-occupations of guilt, and which cannot be relieved by reassurance.

Hallucinations can be brought on by noises, smells or tastes. Hearing may become highly acute with some people hearing distant traffic noise not heard by others. Helen Razor captures such nuances in her book *Gas Smells Awful*: 'The tiniest sound can make you start. Music is deafening . . . Taste is repugnant. Mildly offensive smells work your gut into a frenzy. Everything appears to have hideously sharp edges . . . you can smell colour, savour sound, feel invisible objects.'[7]

In such severe states of depression, many people feel a 'burden' on others and may seek to kill themselves or, if they feel that 'the whole world is a burden', may kill others to protect them. This explains the rare but tragic situation of a post-natal 'puerperal psychosis' (see pages 40–1), where a caring mother may kill or harm her baby.

☆ Coping repertoires in bipolar disorder

> . . . an illness that is biological in its origins, yet one feels psychological in the experience of it.
>
> Kay Jamison, *An Unquiet Mind*

People with bipolar disorder generally get both 'highs' and 'lows' (although a small number get only 'highs'). The 'lows' are almost always of the melancholic depressive 'type'.

During the 'high', the individual feels terrific and is very confident. Talk is increased and is so much faster than usual that others seem unable to keep up. The mind races with ideas, and creativity is distinctly increased—certainly in the mind of the individual, but often in reality too. People with bipolar disorder have lots of energy and need less sleep than usual— perhaps getting up in the middle of the night to do housework, or write 'The Great Australian Novel'! Sexual interest (and activity) commonly increase. Dressing is often more colourful, and singing more common. The world looks brighter and more attractive (trees are greener, water more sparkling). However, as the world is seen through 'rose-coloured glasses' judgment may be poor. Purchases, loans, affairs and other commitments can be undertaken without due regard for the consequences.

While those with depression risk dropping in the social hierarchy, those in a manic or hypomanic mood may rise in the hierarchy. For instance, the shy schoolgirl may ask the captain of the rugby team to take her to the school dance and behave that night with complete self-confidence. Others may persuasively ask for a salary rise, or propose to 'Miss Impossible' and, at times, succeed.

Although highs can make most people feel happy, friendly and amusing, as with alcohol, others can become irritable and aggressive. Experiencing bipolar disorder is as if your brakes have failed; whatever direction you are going in—whether gambling, shopping, driving, having sex, drinking, taking drugs or showing off—you are going too far and too fast.

Kay Jamison has described her high:[8]

> . . . everything seemed so easy. I raced about like a crazed weasel, bubbling with plans and enthusiasms . . . I felt great. Not just great, I felt *really* great. I felt I could do anything, that no task was too difficult . . . not only did everything make perfect sense, but it all began to fit into a marvellous kind of cosmic relatedness.

Of course, there are some advantages in experiencing a high and a lot may be achieved as a result. Many of the world's top creative people have suffered bipolar disorder. But it is an 'asset' with liabilities. If most people were said to have four-cylinder brains, people with bipolar disorder have V8s. Unfortunately, they also have cheap drum brakes. Quite a dangerous combination!

7

Post-natal mood disorders

The adjustments required for a new baby mean that most parents experience some stress and certainly experience many common features of depression, including sleep deprivation, low energy and social withdrawal. The increased stress will certainly lead to a higher level of anxiety in most parents. The boundary between 'normal' adjustment functioning and the less severe post-natal disorders can be somewhat blurred.

As with the depressive disorders, there is no single condition of 'post-natal depression'. Instead, there is a range of conditions, the principal ones briefly summarised below.

☆ Maternity blues

Most women experience normal mood changes but following the birth of a child these usually settle within the second week. So-called 'maternity blues' are therefore relatively normal, and are likely to be caused by an extreme reduction in hormone levels (of both oestrogen and progesterone) immediately post-partum, showing a rather similar mechanism to premenstrual mood shifts. Only a minority of women, even those with severe 'maternity blues', go on to develop a formal post-natal depressive disorder.

☆ Post-natal depression

Post-natal depression refers to a clinical depressive disorder occurring within the first six months after the birth of a baby.

The overall incidence is held to be about 1 in 10, but this 10 per cent may be somewhat inflated by inclusion of conditions other than clinical depression (especially anxiety disorders). The chance of clinical depression occurring during this period is approximately three times the overall new episode rate for depression in women over their lifetime. Most post-natal depressive states are non-melancholic in type, but show depressive features akin to that condition. They commonly involve a focus of fears, depressive ruminations and obsessions about the wellbeing of the baby, as well as the woman's perceived inadequacy as a mother. A significant number of women have fears of harming their baby.

For those who are genetically or otherwise biologically predisposed to develop melancholic depression, the post-natal period is a high-risk time for developing the condition, whether as an initial episode or as a recurrence. It is uncommon for a new episode of melancholic depression to commence during pregnancy.

☆ Puerperal psychosis

Puerperal psychosis is an all-encompassing term used to describe any psychotic condition occurring in the first month post-partum. The psychotic features of depression (delusions and hallucinations) are usually extremely florid and therefore very disturbing to the woman and to family members. In addition, the woman may appear quite cognitively affected— that is, in terms of being aware of what is happening to her. A small percentage of women may have a first onset or a recurrence of a schizophrenic episode but, over the last few decades, we have come to realise that the majority of such episodes are primary mood disorders. Thus, the post-partum period provides a distinctly increased risk for those women who are genetically disposed to develop bipolar disorder or melancholic depression. The main features of the depression are manic episodes, psychotic depressive episodes and, quite commonly, mixed states where both manic and depressive features are experienced. Onset is usually sudden, within the first two or three weeks after the birth of the baby. While the episodes are florid and disturbing at the time, the outcome is usually good with most women responding well to treatment. There is, however, an increased suicide risk for women during the first year of treatment.

Treatment options for the clinical condition are considered in more detail later, but there are some specific features to take into account when dealing with a diagnosis of post-natal depression. A family history of depression or previous episodes of depression increase the chance of a woman developing a post-natal mood disorder, as do a number of psychosocial factors including low self-esteem, exposure to poor parenting practices, or difficulties with a spouse.

Management of post-natal depression should involve assessment by trained primary health care staff such as early childhood or mothercraft nurses, or antenatal midwives, all of whom have the experience to know when to provide management themselves and when to refer women for medical or psychiatric assessment.

Drug treatment during pregnancy and while breastfeeding is clearly an extremely important issue in terms of the health of the baby. General principles suggest that if a woman is on antidepressant or mood stabilising medication, consultation with an expert should be undertaken and drug-free conception attempted. In the first three months of pregnancy certain medications should be avoided but this cannot always be done. In such cases, the mother, her partner and her doctor have to work together to address cost-benefit issues. (See the references on page 139 to the work of Dr Austin and Professor Mitchell who provide details on the effects of pyschotropic drugs.)

8

Grief: the experience

Grief differs considerably from depression. In depression, there is a drop in self-esteem and self-worth. In grief, there is either internal distress over the loss of another, or external distress over the loss of an ideal. When grief is at its worst, such distress is usually experienced as overwhelming separation anxiety.

Grief is generally experienced in stages. The first stage, which may last from hours to days, is a phase of 'numbness' where the individual is in a state of disbelief or even denial. The second stage, which may last from weeks to several months, is when separation anxiety is at its most severe as waves of grief, sadness and tears are experienced. During this stage, sleep and appetite disturbances are common, as are social withdrawal, a sense of guilt or a wish to blame others. The lost individual may be 'seen' or experienced in some way. The third stage, which may commence after weeks or months, is associated with a cessation of social withdrawal, a settling of distressful symptoms and the return of happy or positive memories of the dead individual. Only one-third of grieving people actually go on to develop distinct depression, but usually not until weeks or months after their loss.

This biphasic response of grief (first phase) and depression (second phase) may be a 'built in' response designed to promote survival. An analogy from the animal kingdom will make the argument clearer. Imagine a mother and infant monkey in the jungle. The mother disappears and, after an interval, the baby begins to emit high-pitched screams and run around in a seemingly erratic way. If it is not reunited with its mother, the infant is likely to assume a fixed, slumped over, immobile position. Why?

The first phase is designed to re-establish contact with the mother. Assuming that she has just wandered away, she is more likely to see a darting infant, hear its screams, and come running back. If, however, the mother has been taken by a predator, it would be unwise for the infant to continue such behaviours—even if it were not taken by the same predator, it would soon become exhausted. The second phase of behaviour therefore protects the infant against both detection and dehydration or heat loss. In other words, first-phase anxiety is designed to promote re-attachment, while second-phase 'depression' promotes survival.

Thus, grief (separation anxiety) is a state distinct from depression (loss), although it may lead to a depressive state.

The following example illustrates a situation in which it is difficult to determine where grief ends and depression begins, as the two states seem to overlap to such a degree.

A 23-year-old woman states that she became severely distressed when she found that her boyfriend had been unfaithful to her and had left her for the 'other woman'. In the first week she was unable to sleep for more than two or three hours a night, had completely lost her appetite and admitted to a significant weight loss of 6 kg. She was crying repeatedly. She then described being hypervigilant, jumping at any loud noise and on more than one occasion she thought she saw her boyfriend and his red sports car—only to find that it was a complete stranger. She felt insecure, jumpy and anxious. Interestingly, at that time she noted a fantasy of being pregnant. She cannot remember any loss of self-esteem, and was more distressed by the loss of her boyfriend and her sense that they had formed a couple.

In the second week, she observed less anxiety and insecurity and reported that her sleep, although still patchy, was improving, as was her appetite. However, she was then aware, either validly or not, that she had lost her boyfriend irrevocably, and felt hopeless, helpless and depressed. Her self-esteem dropped, she became critical of herself and started blaming herself for having 'lost another bloke'.

In the third week, she stopped going to work or discussing the issue with her girlfriends. Instead, she spent the days lying in bed and pigging out on boxes of chocolates.

This example describes the biphasic process noted earlier, with grief rather than depression being the driving condition in the first week. Her fantasies of pregnancy can be presumed to reflect her wish to be reunited with her boyfriend or, if she couldn't have him, to have at least part of him. It could also signify her desire for a surrogate relationship with another person she could care for—a baby. She moves into depression in the second week. In the third week, she chooses a self-consolatory strategy as a way of dealing with her pain (eating chocolate in response to food cravings). She is 'caring' for herself in a surrogate way, with an unconscious motivation of 'I'll care for myself as I wish to be cared for, as no one else is caring for me'.

Perhaps the most severe examples of a grief–depression sequence are observed in mothers who have had a young baby die, for example, from Sudden Infant Death Syndrome (SIDS). Here the response pattern is so distinct that we can only wonder at how instinctive the behaviour is and the role of evolution. In the first week after the death of the baby the mother might wake during the night and run through the house searching for her baby, even emitting high-pitched screams. After days or weeks, the high arousal pattern is replaced by one in which the mother spends most of her time slumped, rarely responding to others and appearing almost robotic. The depressed state begins to overwhelm her.

The two phases of any biphasic response (that is, high arousal and depression) following a significant loss generally overlap, rather than forming time-discrete stages. This makes it difficult to determine whether an individual's current state is one of grief, depression or a combination of both.

As noted earlier, only one-third of people experiencing grief will go on to develop a distinct depressive phase. Most will experience a range of alternating and evolving grief stages before some resolution occurs.

Grief can be suppressed, unresolved or prolonged. In such cases the grief can be labelled 'pathological'. The commonest causes of unresolved grief are blocked anger or suppressed emotions, and the excessive use of benzodiazepines such as Valium, or other drugs that suppress grief and its processing.

While some antidepressant drugs can reduce the intensity of grief, a range of proven counselling techniques is generally preferred to medication.

9

Personality styles and non-melancholic depression

The influence of personality on melancholic depression and psychotic melancholia is, at best, slight and may even be non-existent. Personality and temperament appear to be of relevance only to the non-melancholic disorders. (Temperament can be best defined as 'hard-wired' and largely genetically driven. Personality, on the other hand, can be defined as temperament modified by life situations generally experienced in our early years.)

There are a number of temperament and personality 'styles' that are commonly represented in non-melancholic depression. Those suffering from this disorder could:

- be anxious, or anxious worriers;
- see themselves as shy;
- have a low self-esteem or sense of self-worth;
- be controlling and perfectionist (and become vulnerable when they lose control or have it taken away);
- be sensitive to, or expect rejection in, social and close relationships;
- be volatile and both frustrated and impatient when their needs are not met.

It is important to remember that not all clinically observed personality styles actually increase the individual's chance of developing depression. Indeed, some actually decrease the chance of depression. For example, while some people who develop a non-melancholic depression have an 'obsessional' personality, 'obsessionality' is actually somewhat protective, so that 'obsessional' people are less likely to become depressed. A second example involves those with a volatile, impulsive and reckless personality style that may dispose them to depression, but also lead to rapid resolution because they 'externalise' their distress.

Thus, here, we are not considering 'at-risk' personality styles (that is, ones that necessarily increase the chance of clinical depressive episodes), but more ones that trigger and shape the non-melancholic depressive disorder and which need to be factored into any treatment or management plan.

Models of so-called 'normal temperament' emphasise four principal underpinning dimensions. First, we all range along a dimension of being 'anxious worriers' through to demonstrating immense resilience to stressful events. Second, we range across an introversion versus extroversion dimension, from being shy and preferring our own company to being party animals seeking novelty, stimulation and excitement. Third, in the dimension of task-orientation, we may function from highly reliable, conscientious, work-focused and even perfectionistic through to easygoing, unreliable and even feckless. The fourth dimension is simply described as 'agreeableness', where we range across a gradient of being pleasant and caring to viewing others as being there principally to meet our needs. Some personality styles observed clinically appear to reflect basic temperaments (for example, anxious worrying), while others (such as self-blaming) may be acquired.

As each of these personality and temperament 'styles' is dimensional, it is rare for individuals to be placed at risk of depression in relation to only one. Nevertheless, each of the four dimensions has some relevance. These are some of the personality 'faces' of people who develop non-melancholic depression, with each 'face' not only defining the individual's vulnerability to depressive disorders, but also informing us about how the individual is likely to handle their depression.

The personality style may therefore help shape the therapeutic intervention.

At highest risk of developing non-melancholic depression are those with an 'anxious worrying' personality style. People with this personality type tend to have family members with a similar temperament style (arguing for a genetic contribution). They are at high risk of developing both anxiety and depressive disorders, which frequently appear in adolescence or early adulthood. Why are they so at risk? Simply because worry drives and perpetuates depression. The next at-risk group is those who have an ongoing low self-worth and who blame themselves when things go wrong. They often turn early criticism into self-criticism and depression.

The third at-risk group is those who are shy and introverted. This group tends to remember themselves in their younger years as being reserved, with few or no friends, and generally avoiding social interaction and being inhibited in their behaviours toward others. As might be predicted, there is an overlap between anxious worriers and the shy and introverted, with anxious worriers likely to remember themselves as being shy in childhood.

The fourth group comprises those who rate high on reliability and conscientiousness, and who are highly self-controlled. They control their environment in direct and indirect ways so as to reduce the chance of being exposed to stressful events. This group is also less likely to seek clinical attention as doing so would involve a risk of surrendering control—a central issue of concern. They are, however, most likely to develop depression when they have lost 'control' of an issue that they see as their responsibility (such as their child not taking up an expected career choice or getting into a relationship judged to be unsatisfactory). This group are highly valued as community members, and we seek them out to be our doctors, lawyers or financial advisers. Their vulnerability is the flip-side to their personality style—they lack flexibility and are less adroit in situations when they are required to move from an entrenched view. Their sense of pride—not only in their work but in many other matters—also leaves them particularly vulnerable to depression (and even to suicide) when their reputation or judgment is challenged or impugned.

These four groups can all be described as having 'internalising' personality styles. When stressed, they tend to go quiet, muse and worry and retreat from others. Their stress and depression is experienced at the emotional and cognitive level.

This is in sharp contrast to those who have a more 'externalising' personality style, of which there are two common types. With the first type, the individual externalises anxiety as irritability when stressed and often becomes irritated by little things, is rattled easily, is quick-tempered and quite 'snappy'. With the second type, the individual tends to be dramatic, emotional, volatile and often erratic in their general functioning. As the psychiatrist Kay Jamison puts it: 'For those with a short wick . . . and impulse-laden wiring, life's setbacks and illness are more dangerous.' [1]

While both personality styles are frequent in those who develop depression, individuals in the second group are less likely to develop persisting clinical non-melancholic depression. They are more likely to externalise their depression by raising their voice, arguing, throwing things or by being reckless. By releasing their frustration and distress in these ways, they often recover rapidly from their depressed mood. Those around them, however, may end up distressed from the fallout. As Jamison notes, for those who are impetuous and volatile, 'their . . . risktaking will make them generators and throwers of sparks as well [as] . . . high-wire acts and dealers in discord'.[2]

While there are many personality styles, most can be considered in reference to the six dimensions just described. For example, 'interpersonal sensitivity' has been held to be a key risk factor in non-melancholic depression. Here individuals tend to avoid others for fear that they will be rejected, disapproved of, ridiculed or criticised. Thus they feel socially inept and inferior to others. Predictably, they rate high on shyness and introversion, the third dimension. Interestingly, when depressed, a percentage of people with interpersonal sensitivity develop a clinical pattern of features that contrast with the usual profile, often describing appetite increase rather than appetite loss, and excessive sleep rather than insomnia. As noted in an earlier chapter, excessive sleeping may restore slow-wave sleep during stressful periods, while food cravings may increase L-tryptophan levels and thus serotonergic transmission. Our research suggests that individuals with interpersonal sensitivity are highly likely to have a primary anxiety disorder. The term **atypical depression** was developed to describe this clinical constellation of depressive and personality features.

A key cognitive theory of depression argues that those who develop depression view themselves, their future and the world in a negative way, and that this view is ongoing. A number of recent research studies, however, have suggested that such views are generally held only when an individual is depressed. Their role in causing depression, therefore, has been downgraded in recent times.

Cognitive theorists quite reasonably argue that it is the way in which we see the world, rather than the way the world actually is, that influences our judgments and may or may not lead to depression. Thus, those who do not believe themselves to be particularly influential or masterful are more likely to develop depression. A related 'locus of control' theory similarly suggests that those who have an 'external locus of control' (that is, they see themselves as a cork on the ocean, prone to being moved around at the whim of others) are highly likely to develop depression. This is in sharp contrast with those who have a strong 'internal locus of control'; that is, they view themselves as masters of their own destiny and have their hand on the tiller.

☆ Clinical presentation of personality styles

Under stress, personality styles can be magnified. Clinicians see three common patterns in individuals who present with a non-melancholic depression—in addition to many rare and even unique ones. Most common are patterns of (i) anxious worrying, (ii) declared irritability, or manifest volatility, anger and even hostility, and (iii) evident long-standing low self-confidence and high self-blame.

Anxious worriers are highly likely to have had a clinical anxiety disorder (such as panic disorder, social phobia or obsessive compulsive disorder) before developing their initial depressive episode. Where an individual is both depressed and irritable or hostile, two sub-groups appear to exist. Those in the first sub-group are intrinsically anxious (and generally do not have a volatile personality). They become more anxious with their depressive episode, and then externalise their anxiety via irritability. The second sub-group is made up of those who have an ongoing volatile personality style and who generally become angered when their needs are not met.

The third pattern has been defined as a 'depressive personality' style by some writers. It describes those whose usual mood is gloomy and unhappy, whose self-concept is dominated by beliefs of inadequacy and low self-esteem, and who are often self-critical and negative. Such people often report life-long depression. 'Depression' may be little more than an extension of these long-standing characteristics, so that people in the third group often have difficulty in determining when episodes start and finish.

How can we make better sense of these differing clinical profiles which reflect a mixture of personality styles and depressive features? What are the processes that lie behind the different classes? While personality and temperament styles contribute to non-melancholic depression in many ways, a key factor is their influence on emotional equilibrium.

☆ Emotional equilibrium

Emotional equilibrium is a state of stable balance, such that any disturbance from outside tends to be corrected.

Let's assume that everyone has an internal 'regulating machine' that requires 'resetting' after an upsetting event. Most people will develop a depressed mood after an upsetting event, but the great majority return to emotional equilibrium within days (that is, they have a 'normal' depressed mood state). Some people, however, are unable to reset their mechanism easily, thus losing their 'emotional equilibrium'. They remain essentially 'stuck'. Their personality styles and ways of dealing with events 'sustain' the depression, rather than enabling them to 'get over it'.

So how can equilibrium be lost? There are two main ways:

1. The machinery can fail; for example, if the keel on a yacht breaks off, the yacht will capsize.
2. A 'positive feedback loop' can develop. This means that two or more factors can influence each other to such a degree that a small disturbance leads to a further disturbance. This loop is sometimes also called a 'vicious circle'. An example of feedback occurs when a microphone is put too close to a speaker. A small noise from the speaker is amplified into the mike, and further amplified by the speaker. While the feedback loop can be of use to create musical effects, such reverberation (mulling over and rumination) is not useful for humans.

☆ Conclusion

Non-melancholic depressions represent what happens when an upsetting event occurs to people with personality styles that 'sustain' depression. Those with internalising personalities may create internal feedback. They stew on and worry about the upsetting event, become increasingly self-critical, and keep the mental image of the problem humming round their circuits. They operate like a feedback loop. Those with externalising personalities may 'sustain' their depression by over-reacting to a disturbance and generating new incoming drama, a bit like a guitarist standing close to a loud amplifier.

In addition to treating the depression, the management of non-melancholic depression requires consideration to be given as to how the predisposing and sustaining personality characteristics (such as worrying, irritability, self-critical talk, volatility) can be modified to achieve greater emotional equilibrium. If non-melancholic depression is to be effectively treated, the personality contribution that can both dispose to, and maintain, depressive episodes needs to be identified and modified.

10

Stress and depressive sub-types

It is possible that an individual's episode of depression may be caused entirely by a major stressful situation or event. For others, stressors may 'set off' or trigger an episode that was 'waiting to happen'. Alternatively, a depressive episode may be completely unrelated to a stressful event. It is therefore not surprising that, in many written accounts of depression, the role of stressful events as a trigger is difficult to determine. Often, the explanations provided by therapists are just as speculative.

In conjunction with other identified risk factors, this chapter will look at two broad groups of stressful events—distal events, which may have occurred years previously, and proximal events, which occur close to the onset a depressive disorder.

☆ Distal stressors

Some distal risk factors are biological (for example, genetic influences, brain damage from injury or alcohol abuse). Many act to increase social risk and appear to have particular relevance to the non-melancholic disorders. Sex (or gender) is a good example. A consistent finding from studies of normal communities is that women are more likely to develop depression than men, although bipolar disorder and melancholia have similar lifetime rates in men and women. This would seem to suggest an over-representation of non-melancholic depression in women, and could indicate the 'anxious worrying' (see page 51) style being more common in women. In groups where there is social homogeneity (for example, where men and women have the same occupations) the difference between men and women is so slight as to be non-existent (as established by Mood Disorders Unit Researcher, Professor Wilhelm). Anatomy is therefore not necessarily destiny.

The type of parenting received can also be a distal stressor. Low levels of care and lack of affection from a parent increase the chance of depression, as does exposure to a parent who is controlling and overprotective. Low levels of parental care may make the child insecure—acting as a direct stressor—which in turn can lead to a child developing a low sense of self-worth. This creates a vulnerability in the adult to stressful events that reflect on self-esteem. A controlling parent often effectively delays a child's normal progress to independence, with the result that the child is later ill-equipped to handle the everyday tasks required of adult life. This, in turn, makes the adult easily stressed and more likely to develop depression when faced with adverse events.

Socioeconomic levels can also act as distal stressors. The lower the social class in the early years, the greater the chance of non-melancholic depression in adulthood—presumably because of increased exposure to a range of stressful factors. Social class does not appear to have any clear relationship to melancholic depression, although bipolar disorder appears to be somewhat over-represented in higher social class groups.

Most of the distal social stressors that dispose a person to non-melancholic depression are, however, modifiable. For example, someone exposed to uncaring parenting will be at much less risk of developing depression if they subsequently have a caring partner who can act in a 'buffer' role, or who can modify the risk elements. Conversely, someone who has experienced caring parenting but is then demeaned by their spouse, is more likely to develop depression than someone who has experienced only caring relationships.

☆ Proximal stressors

Proximal stressful events are the presumed 'causes' of depression. Some, such as substance abuse (excessive intake of alcohol or drugs, both prescribed and illegal), are more influential than generally conceded.

In non-melancholic disorders, depression is much more a consequence of an interaction between an immediate stressor and the individual's temperament and personality style. The same stressful event can evoke a wide range of responses in different people. Some may ignore it, others worry about it. Some may feel that 'all is lost' and others that the ability to control life has slipped away. The individual's reaction to the stressor contributes to both the onset of the depression and its severity.

The most common causes of melancholic, psychotic and bipolar depression appear 'biological'. In the past, melancholic depression was called 'endogenous' depression, meaning coming from 'within'. It was therefore considered to be independent of stress. However, stress may precipitate a biological reaction, thus bringing on depression. (A number of medical conditions, for example diabetes, can be similarly brought on by stress in those predisposed to the disease.) As the melancholic disorders are more likely to commence from the age of 40 onwards, an 'age effect' on the brain must be conceded. Some external factors may be relevant for the more biological disorders. For example, in comparison to non-melancholic disorders, the onset of manic, psychotic and melancholic depressive episodes is increased in spring, indicating a seasonal cause. The rapid increase in hours of bright sunshine is thought to trigger depression and mania by affecting the pineal gland.

It does seem that the principal depressive sub-types show

varying susceptibility (or resistance) to certain life stresses. This idea is developed further on the following pages.

How does 'stress' lead to depression in the non-melancholic disorders?

The Mood Disorders Unit suspects that non-melancholic disorders are primarily caused by psychological processes reflecting an interaction between stress and the individual's personality. A central feature of 'depression' is loss of one's self-esteem (that is, thinking less of oneself or being increasingly self-critical). Any event, therefore, that impacts on an individual's sense of self-worth risks precipitating depression.

A common stress event to impact on self-esteem is the break-up of an intimate relationship. The event itself is irrelevant—it is the individual's response to the event that is crucial. Consider an individual who responds to a marital break-up with, 'My wife has left me for another man as she thinks I'm a jerk, and everything recently just confirms what a hopeless human being I am.' Contrast this with somebody who says, 'My wife—what a jerk—has left me. Great. I can get on with life again.' The chance of developing depression is greater for the first respondent than the second. This is because the event differed in terms of its impact on each individual's self-esteem levels or because they 'processed' the event differently as a result of their differing personalities.

Stressful events can be acute (a marital break-up) or ongoing (a dysfunctional marriage), but both have an impact on an individual's self-esteem.

Many people who develop a non-melancholic disorder have such a low ongoing self-image, or their personality type is such, that any stressful event is likely to trigger depression. In a sense, some people actually create their own triggers. For example, a woman who thinks that everyone rejects her may misinterpret a remark at a party and become immediately and distinctly depressed.

How does 'stress' lead to depression in melancholic and psychotic depression?

The brain is made up of anatomical sections and numerous circuits (the latter like railroad tracks). If, for example, the **basal ganglia** (the brain centres refining motor performance) and the **pre-frontal cortex** (a structural region at the front of the brain) are disrupted, there are three principal effects: depressed mood, observable PMD and cognitive problems.

Disruption of these circuits can occur in response to stress or even spontaneously. We can presume that certain neurotransmitters (these modulate mood and other mental states) have been 'turned off'. Many factors may influence neurotransmitter function. In melancholic depression (and, less clearly in psychotic depression) there is often a family history of depression, suggesting a genetic influence. People with melancholic depression will commonly report a significant stress prior to their first, or first few, episodes. Subsequent episodes tend to appear more spontaneously and are less clearly related to stressful events. Therefore, certain genetic influences may create a vulnerability that initially requires a stress event to trigger the depressive state.

Physics provides a useful analogy with Hookes' Law, which states that if elastic objects are stretched within their limitations, they will 'bounce back' to their previous state. If, however, they are stretched beyond a certain point, their elasticity is lost. In melancholic depression, for example, it seems that initial elasticity allows the vulnerable individual to be unaffected by stressful events—for a period at least. However, once a formal episode has occurred, the elasticity is lessened and future episodes may occur without the individual being 'stretched' or 'stressed'. Vulnerability has been manifested and is no longer latent.

Certain drugs and some diseases can also act like environmental stressors, in that they have the capacity to disrupt some of the brain's neural circuits linking the basal ganglia and pre-frontal cortex (presumably by using differing pathways and affecting mechanisms). In older people, the effects of the aging brain may disrupt the circuits in other ways. There are parallels between these depressive conditions and Parkinson's disease (which causes changes in the basal ganglia and other parts of the brain), including depression and a movement disorder. These parallels provide some understanding of biological depressive disorders such as melancholia. In psychotic melancholia, the disruptions in the brain's circuitry are more severe and extend to other brain circuits and regions, causing delusions and hallucinations as well as severe PMD.

☆ A metaphor on the road

There was a neuronal pileup on the highways of my brain, and the more I tried to slow down my thinking the more I became aware that I couldn't. My enthusiasms were going into overdrive . . .

K. Jamison, *An Unquiet Mind*

This overview of stressors suggests quite different principal causes and factors relating to the different depressive types, with distinctive contributions from a range of variables. In all depressive types, stress may have been experienced before an episode, but the stress event itself may or may not have been the determinant, a contributing factor or even a mere non-causal 'after-the-event' interpretation.

An analogy illuminates some of the issues underpinning the key personality 'types' and the varying relevance of life event stress to the broad depressive types. Imagine a busy main road. People cycle along it to get to work. Large trucks also use the road, often travelling at speed. Sometimes they travel very close to the cyclists. A number of cyclists have fallen off and the traffic police have asked why. All the cyclists gave the same response: 'A truck came too close to me and blew me off.'

Further investigations, however, showed that, despite all citing the same reason for their accidents, the cyclists differed from those who didn't fall in quite definite ways.

The non-melancholic cyclists were of two main personality types: internalising and externalising. The internalising non-melancholic cyclists, being inclined to anxious worrying, rode very slowly and cautiously. When a truck passed, they wobbled badly. Their slow speed meant that they had little equilibrium and therefore often hit the kerb.

On the other hand, the externalising non-melancholic cyclists rode rather too fast for safety. They got very angry at any truck that came too close—yelling their irritation, and taking their hands off the handlebars to gesture. Their over-reaction was what upset their equilibrium.

The melancholic depressive, psychotic melancholic and bipolar cyclists had all bought their bikes from the same shop and there were some individual design quirks that made these bikes more demanding to ride.

The melancholic cyclists could travel along quite well, but if they encountered a truck and had to pull onto the road's shoulder, the loose gravel tended to deflate their tyres. Their bikes could only go a short distance before losing momentum, at which point the rider fell off.

When the psychotic melancholic cyclists swerved, the action sheared off a bolt that detached the front wheel! They were no longer able to direct their cycles.

The bipolar cyclists' faulty bikes had gears that sometimes got stuck either in the 'low' or 'high' range. In addition, the brakes were not powerful enough for such high performance machines. Any swerve to avoid a truck exposed this instability, though their bicycles were difficult to control even in good conditions.

The rest of the cyclists on the road were unaffected by trucks, although some wobbled a bit, but didn't fall off. Many didn't even notice the heavy traffic.

This metaphor explains that internalising personalities may

benefit from therapies that both reduce anxiety and mute their tendency to worry excessively or be insufficiently assertive. Externalising personalities may benefit from learning damage control when faced with a stressful event. For the other types of depression, physical treatments such as medication are almost invariably required to address intrinsic physical debilities.

The suggestion, therefore, is that for certain depressive sub-types there is a 'structural' problem. Some people resist such an interpretation, whereas others are relieved by it (for example, 'I'm sick of being told that I just need to pull up my socks . . . I know I've got a structural problem and I want others to accept it.') The bottom line is that suffering biological depression such as melancholic or bipolar depression is similar to suffering from a medical condition such as diabetes. This reality is unfortunately warped by the stigma that has long distorted and distracted consideration of mental illnesses.

11

Four vignettes

The four vignettes that follow consider the role of biological, social and other factors in depression.

Sue had been a shy and somewhat conservative child. She was 24 when her mother first took her to a psychiatrist, but had had depressive episodes since early adolescence. After losing a job she became increasingly withdrawn. She was anxious, worried, and afraid to go out of the house. She was also tearful, and would frequently retreat to her room and stay in bed, asking her family to say she wasn't home if a friend phoned.

Her family thought she had something on her mind, but she wouldn't tell them what it was. Instead she 'stewed' on her own. Sometimes they would find her crying. Normally very reliable, she was now letting responsibilities lapse, but felt guilty at the same time for letting her family down.

Sue told the doctor that she had avoided relationships to escape being criticised. She had just been 'dropped' by her first boyfriend, so life wasn't worth living. Her normal worrying style had been blown out of all proportion.

Catherine was brought into hospital by her husband, Bob. He said that in recent weeks she had been behaving as she had after the birth of their son, twenty years earlier. Although they had eagerly awaited the baby, after the birth Catherine had become so deeply depressed that she was unable to look after her son. There had been one other episode of depression since then, but it had lifted after some time on antidepressant medication.

She had been going through menopause, and Bob had at first thought that this was the reason for her constant tears and withdrawal. She said that she had no energy and, even though she was tired, she could not sleep through the night. She was lethargic, moved slowly and hardly spoke. Formerly an excellent hostess, she had stopped contacting friends, and lost both her interest in cooking and her appetite.

Bob found her late one night with a bottle of tablets and, although she assured him that she wouldn't harm herself, she confessed that she had been thinking what a relief it would be to be dead.

Jason was normally an extrovert, always on the go, moving from one interest to another and needing a lot of stimulation. He was the life of the party, eager to meet people and warming quickly to new friendships. He had had a number of relationships, but was a bit fickle. He would fall intensely in love, but then find his partner boring after a while.

He became depressed after losing his job, a consequence of a few too many 'sickies'. He started to take his frustrations out on his girlfriend, snapping at her constantly. He also got into arguments with his family.

He told his doctor that he was aware of how irritable he had become and, while he regretted it, he said he couldn't control his feelings. He had recently smashed a DVD player to 'let off some steam'. It had made him feel somewhat better, temporarily.

Harry, a 67-year-old widower, was admitted to hospital after a concerned neighbour and his general practitioner had found him unkempt and very agitated.

In hospital he initially refused food, saying that his insides had rotted away. Preoccupied and distressed by this delusion, he was unable to be reassured by the staff. He paced constantly, wringing his hands and saying over and over, 'What will become of me?'

He told staff that he was being punished for his failures and indiscretions. His guilt was out of proportion to the incidents he then described: for instance, he felt he deserved to go to jail for failing to include a minor payment on his tax return twenty years ago.

A relative remembered that Harry had been like this before, once soon after he had returned from the war, and twice in the last few years. One episode came on after Harry thought he had sped through a police radar. He was convinced that this incident had caused his depression. An uncle had been hospitalised for a similar setback.

In the absence of specific markers for melancholic and psychotic depression, both Sue and Jason are more likely to have a non-melancholic depression. Sue's symptoms are indicative of an 'internalising' personality style, while Jason's are of an 'externalising' style, with both those styles contributing to the onset and persistence of the depression.

On the other hand, Catherine's and Harry's depressions appear more biologically based, with psychomotor disturbance (retardation and agitation respectively) evident. Harry is also experiencing psychotic episodes. Catherine is likely to have melancholic depression and Harry, with his delusions, a psychotic melancholia. Their depressions appear unrelated to personality style with the biological stressors hormonal in Catherine's case and genetic in Harry's.

However, it should be noted that determining depressive 'type' on the basis of family history, 'biological' stressors, personality style or a single stressful event is limited. Instead, diagnostic sub-typing should be driven by looking for type-specific clinical features such as psychomotor disturbance and evidence of psychosis.

12

The biology of depression

While our knowledge of the working brain is still limited, in most instances of clinical depression it is likely that neurotransmitter function is disrupted. Another term for neurotransmission is 'nerve conduction', but what does this mean?

The human brain contains about 100 billion neurones, or nerve cells, which are a bit like tiny wires. Wires in a TV are joined together by solder, but the brain's wires are joined by junctions called 'synapses'. A signal from one part of the brain to another travels as a series of electrical impulses along a neurone until it reaches a synapse. At that point the synapse releases a tiny speck of a chemical, a 'neurotransmitter', which jumps the gap in the synapse and lands on the surface of the next neurone, so passing on information from nerve cell to nerve cell. In normal brain function, the signal is as strong in the second and subsequent neurones as it was in the first.

Figure 12.1   Neurotransmitters and the functioning of the brain

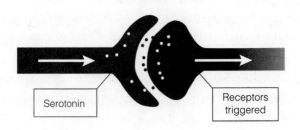

There are thought to be many different neurotransmitters in the brain for many different purposes, one of which is undoubtedly mood regulation. So far, about 100 have been identified, including serotonin. Serotonin is known to be involved in three important circuits: sleep, mood and aggression, and pain control. It is likely that in most causes of depression (especially non-melancholic depression), serotonergic transmission in the brain is less active, and there is less serotonin available in the synapse to stimulate the flow of information from neurone to neurone. Lowered levels of serotonin are associated with depression and suicidal behaviour, as well as with impulsive and aggressive behaviours.

Figure 12.2   **Serotonin neurotransmission in certain types of depression**

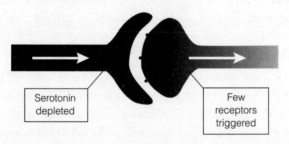

Serotonin depleted

Few receptors triggered

It is likely that in melancholic and psychotic depression other neurotransmitters such as noradrenaline and dopamine fail to function normally across differing regions of the brain. It is clear, therefore, that the extent to which different neurotransmitters and varying circuits are involved contributes to the principal sub-types of depression. This has ramifications for the effectiveness of the various classes of antidepressant drugs and other physical treatments such as electroconvulsive therapy, transcranial magnetic stimulation and mood stabilisers.

☆ What's the solution?

As noted in Chapter 10, causes and triggers of depression can operate at different levels. These are:

- biological (for example, genetic, the effects of drugs and/or specific medical problems);
- psychological (for example, low self-esteem, personality style); and
- social (for example, distressing life events, dysfunctional relationship).

Solutions, too, can be considered at biological, psychological and social levels.

Biological solutions

Any biological treatment must involve the correct identification of the principal depressive sub-type. For psychotic and melancholic depression, the primary treatment solution is generally physical (such as antidepressant drugs), whereas for many of the non-melancholic disorders the primary treatment is more likely to be psychosocial.

Treatments, however, are not always linked to causes. One wise psychiatrist noted that 'migraine is not caused by an insufficiency of aspirin'. A significant percentage of the non-melancholic depressive disorders respond to antidepressant medications, and, while a patient with a melancholic depression may respond well to an antidepressant drug, secondary issues might be best dealt with using an alternative approach (for example, counselling for marital problems).

A pluralistic or integrated approach may also be of benefit. Assuming that an individual's depression is being maintained by low levels of serotonin in the brain, then alternative therapies (not all conclusively proved to date) might involve some of the suggestions listed below.

Imagine all the synapses as leaky rain tanks running low on serotonin. The obvious solution is to find a way of refilling the tanks. This could be done by turning off the tap or by mending the leak.

Turning off the tap. This means, stop doing anything that is contributing to the problem. For example:

- address the trigger that caused the problem;
- sleep where you are unlikely to be disturbed;
- check whether any medication you are on can cause depression;
- get any thyroid or other medical problem treated;
- avoid caffeine as it contributes to insomnia and anxiety;
- as far as possible avoid major life changes or dramas;
- avoid alcohol and illicit drugs;
- treat chronic pain;
- declare a truce in major conflicts; and
- don't take up smoking.

Mending the leak. Stop the drain of serotonin and other neurotransmitters from the synapses by using an appropriate antidepressant medication. This may not only alleviate the depression but may also modify an 'at-risk' personality style (for example, 'anxious worrying' or 'irritability') thus increasing resistance to future depressive episodes.

Psychological solutions

Psychological treatments aim to support and counsel the individual during the depressive episode, as well as generate resistance to future episodes by increasing self-esteem and modifying at risk personality styles. Cognitive Behavioural Therapy (CBT) and Interpersonal Therapy (IPT) are the most common formalised approaches (detailed in Chapters 16 and 17).

Social solutions

Social interventions aim to decrease the occurrence and impact of stressful events and promote the socialisation of the individual. The depressed person is encouraged to take part in pleasant activities, counteracting any tendency to shun social contact and thus maintain the depression. A shy individual may be encouraged to develop a repertoire of socialising strategies (through social skills training) or to use assertiveness training to become more self-assured. 'Social engineering' approaches are also relevant here; for example, encouraging someone in a dysfunctional relationship or work environment to make changes that will boost self-esteem.

13

Professional assessment

You just can't seem to get good help these days.

Helen Razor, *Gas Smells Awful*

Most people with depression consult a professional willingly but some, particularly adolescents, may have to be forcefully encouraged or even coerced by others. People who are in this position should inform the professional that they are presenting 'under sufferance' and then establish the 'rules' that will apply to the relationship. Minors may be concerned that the assessment procedure will result in information being passed on to their parents, and adults may worry that their case will be discussed with their spouse.

Professionals have an obligation to respect confidences. Any concerns about how the interview data will be recorded, or who will have access to it, should be raised at the start of the interview. If the professional is able to provide reassurance about patient confidentiality, the patient should try to face the assessment with an open mind.

It is becoming more common for patients to bring a family member or friend to an assessment interview. In this case, the professional must establish whether the patient wants to be interviewed alone or with the other person present. It is usually the patient's call; rarely will the professional make the decision. It may be best to start the assessment alone, as this gives the patient more control over private issues. A family member or friend can be invited to join at a later stage, to give their own observations and to be involved in the development of the patient's management plan.

If, however, you are a relative or a friend of someone with depression, the rules are less clear and guidelines are more difficult to draw up. If you are encouraging someone to see a psychiatrist, do not disguise the issue. Do not wait until the day of the appointment before telling them about it. Do not tell them that the appointment is with a 'doctor' or a 'counsellor' if it is with a psychiatrist.

If it is unlikely that your relative will tell the doctor or counsellor of any risks their disorder may pose, such as self-harm, inform the professional or their secretary/reception-ist directly of your concerns. If your relative or friend has a very severe disorder such as psychotic depression or mania, try to accompany them to the appointment. If you are not requested to be present during the initial assessment, ask that you are at least briefed about the management plan. Ideally, however, you should be present while the management plan is being discussed as this will prevent or limit miscommunication, and you may have valuable contributions to make to its development.

☆ What a detailed assessment might cover

At the initial assessment the following questions might be expected to be asked:

- Is depression the principal disorder, or is it secondary to some other condition (for example, anxiety or substance abuse) that should be assessed and treated?
- If depression is the principal disorder, what are its key features (in order to determine the depressive sub-type)?
- What is the risk, if any, to the patient of self-harm, harm to reputation, or even harm to others?
- What is the level of current disability?
- Were there any triggers (for example, stressful events) to the episode?

- If there were triggers, did they entirely cause the depressive state, did they activate or worsen it, or were they merely coincidental?
- How did the patient interpret the triggers, and what thoughts did they activate?
- Is the patient part of a family network and, if so, what is the quality of the relationships?
- What can the patient remember about their childhood, including the level of parenting received, their interactions with other children and their experiences at school?
- Is there any family history of depression or other relevant medical problems?
- How many and what types of jobs has the patient had and what level of satisfaction, if any, was there?
- What is the quality of the patient's relationships with intimates, peers, work mates?   Have those relationships been sustained over time?

The professional should also seek to establish:

- the patient's personality style and repertoire of coping responses, identifying particularly any **cognitive style** that may increase the patient's vulnerability;
- a drug and alcohol history;
- any medical/surgical problems, in particular any that may have contributed to the depression;
- whether or not the patient suffers from any allergies, especially to medication;
- any cognitive limitations affecting concentration, memory and intellectual functioning;
- the patient's life history of depressive episodes, previous treatments and perceived effectiveness or ineffectiveness of these treatments;
- any current 'sustaining' factors to the depression—for example, ongoing work problems or dysfunctional relationships; and

- the patient's own views about the reasons for their depression, and their preferred treatments.

☆ What the patient should be told

Just watch out for One Solution Fits All doctors.

Helen Razor, *Gas Smells Awful*

If the outcome of the assessment is that the patient *is* depressed, then the professional should inform the patient of the diagnosis and identify the likely depressive sub-type. If the patient is suffering from another disorder, for example, anxiety or bipolar disorder, then this should be formally acknowledged. It is important that the professional establish confidence in the diagnosis with the patient.

The professional should also identify to the patient any other problems of significance, as well as any medical or emotional conditions that require investigation and/or treatment. It is important to provide the patient with a pluralistic explanation of why the disorder developed at this particular time. This involves integrating past environmental and developmental factors with genetic influences, stress levels and personality interactions.

The professional should also recommend a management strategy and outline the lines of responsibility for those involved in the case. For example, the general practitioner is to handle X and the non-medical professional to handle Y. The professional should always give the patient an accurate assessment of any costs involved and the likely advantages of the management plan.

Different professionals (psychiatrists, psychologists, general practitioners, nurses, social workers, occupational therapists, counsellors) have different training backgrounds and therapeutic orientations. Their therapeutic approaches may range from the very narrow to the very broad, each having advantages and disadvantages for the management plan.

14

Drug treatments

The most common treatments for depression are drugs. This chapter will look at the three types of drugs used:

- antidepressants;
- tranquillisers; and
- antimanic drugs or 'mood stabilisers'.

☆ Antidepressants

There are several separate families of antidepressants and various antidepressant **drug classes** whose effectiveness ranges across the depressive sub-types. For this reason, antidepressants should not be discounted if one particular type does not work. Even if two antidepressants fail, a careful review should be undertaken. This could show that the patient would benefit from another antidepressant drug, or a combination of drugs.

Although there is no universal method of labelling drugs, antidepressants can be broken down by generation, chemical characteristics and the function of the drug. Drug 'generation' refers to the period of the discovery of the drug and its formal release. Thus, the 'first generation' antidepressants emerged in the late 1950s and were extensively trialled in the 1960s. The second generation antidepressants emerged in the late 1970s and early 1980s, while the third generation drugs have generally been available only during the last decade.

The defining chemical characteristics of the drug classes are determined by their nuclear structure. 'Tricyclic' drugs have a three-ring structure, 'tetracyclic' four, and recently developed 'bicyclic' drugs have a two-ring structure.

The third element underpinning an antidepressant's label refers to the function of the particular drug. For example, drugs that block the enzyme monoamine oxidase (MAO) are subdivided into those that block the enzyme irreversibly (the MAOIs) and those that do so reversibly (the RIMAs). While most antidepressants have multiple actions, many work by inhibiting the reuptake or reabsorption of different neurotransmitters (including serotonin, noradrenaline and dopamine) at the nerve synapses, thus increasing the concentration of that particular neurotransmitter. The first generation antidepressants (the tricyclics and MAOs) act on multiple neurotransmitters. The newer drugs, on the other hand, are more selective in the neurotransmitters they target. This selectivity is captured in the drug class name, such as Selective Serotonin Reuptake Inhibitors (SSRIs).

Are all antidepressants of equal benefit?

Formal trials comparing one drug class against another have allowed many scientific reviewers to conclude that all antidepressants are of equal benefit, and that their differences are due to varying side-effects. The Mood Disorders Unit would argue, however, that the different antidepressants are not of equal benefit. The 'equal benefit' view is largely built on data from drug trials, where relatively 'pure' cases of depression are examined, which are often less severe than those seen in clinical practice. Also, patients with melancholic and psychotic depression are rarely included in clinical trials. When data are collected from 'real world' clinical practice studies, a different picture emerges—one that shows the different classes of antidepressants varying considerably in their effects on the different types of depression.

Table 14.1   Currently available antidepressant drugs

	Drug name
First generation antidepressants	
Tricyclics (TCAs)	Amitriptyline
	Clomipramine
	Dothiepin
	Doxepin
	Imipramine
	Nortriptyline
	Trimipramine
Irreversible Monoamine Oxidaze Inhibitors (MAOIs)	Phenelzine
	Tranylcypromine
Second generation antidepressants	
Tetracyclics	Mianserin
Third generation antidepressants	
Selective Serotonin Reuptake Inhibitors (SSRIs)	Citalopram
	Fluoxetine
	Fluvoxamine
	Paroxetine
	Sertraline
Serotonin and Noradrenaline Reuptake Inhibitors (SNRIs)	Venlafaxine
5-HT2 blockers	Nefazodone
Reversible Inhibitors of Monoamine Oxidase-A (RIMA's)	Moclobemide
Other drug types	
Noradrenaline Reuptake Inhibitor (NARI)	Reboxetine
Dopamine-Noradrenaline Reuptake Inhibitors (DNRIs)	Bupropion
Noradrenergic and Specific Serotonergic Antidepressant (NaSSA)	Mirtazapine

Antidepressants and non-melancholic depression

Some of the newer antidepressants (especially the Selective Serotonin Reuptake Inhibitors, or SSRIs) seem to be equally as effective as the older first-generation antidepressants, may be more readily tolerated in terms of side-effects than the first generation antidepressants and may have beneficial effects beyond treating the depression, for example by decreasing worrying, brooding and irritability.

People with an 'anxious worrier' personality style commonly state that the SSRIs induce a sense of detachment from their problems. The problems are still there, but instead are viewed as if by a non-worrier, so that the individual feels that they are swimming rather than sinking. This means that patients worry less, or for briefer periods, so decreasing the chance of worry developing into a depression. If the patient is already depressed, SSRIs may make the depressive episodes briefer and more manageable. The SSRIs also seem to help a significant percentage of those who externalise their anxiety with bursts of irritability.

Antidepressants and melancholic depression
The older Tricyclics (TCAs) and Irreversible Monoamine Oxidase Inhibitors (MAOIs) appear to be more effective than the SSRIs for melancholic and psychotic depression, but tend to have more side-effects. The effectiveness of a number of the other, newer antidepressants for these depressive sub-types is less clear. Some may be too refined in their action, unlike the first-generation antidepressants, which impact on multiple neurotransmitters. Unfortunately, their impact on multiple neurotransmitters also increases the range of possible side-effects. The first generation antidepressants have also been shown to be more effective in older patients, those who have had multiple episodes, and when PMD is severe.

It would be reasonable for an individual with a first episode of melancholic depression to be commenced on an SSRI or a Serotonin and Noradrenaline Reuptake Inhibitor (SNRI). If treatment is successful, it can be recommended for any subsequent episodes. If this first-line treatment fails, then TCAs and MAOIs should be considered.

Antidepressants and psychotic depression
It is generally not enough to treat psychotic depression with antidepressants alone. Most cases of psychotic depression will

require a combination of drug therapies, for example, an antidepressant and a tranquilliser (see pages 80–1). In some cases, electroconvulsive therapy (ECT) may be needed.

Augmentation of antidepressant drugs

The effectiveness of some antidepressants can be increased by the use of adjunctive or augmentation drugs, for example, thyroid hormones or lithium.

There is increasing evidence to suggest that the new 'atypical' antipsychotic drugs may also have augmenting effects on antidepressants, often working rapidly and also being able to be ceased rapidly in many instances. While not investigated formally, the benefits of such augmenting drugs may only be relevant to melancholic and psychotic depression.

How useful is St John's Wort (hypericum) as an antidepressant?

In May 2000, the popular herbal remedy St John's Wort was evaluated as an antidepressant.[1] The evaluation was based on fourteen trials involving over 1400 adults. In eight trials subjects were given St John's Wort or a placebo, while in the other trials St John's Wort and a tricyclic antidepressant. The doses of St John's Wort ranged from 300–1800 mg/day.

'Responders' were defined as those whose condition had improved by 50 per cent or more. The aggregated studies indicated that 38 per cent of those receiving a placebo were responders, compared to 62 per cent of those receiving St John's Wort and 61 per cent receiving the tricyclic antidepressant. Such data would seem to indicate that St John's Wort is an effective antidepressant (being significantly superior to the placebo) and of comparable effectiveness to the tricyclic antidepressants. However, as trials were generally undertaken on those with mild depression, St John's Wort is likely to be of possible assistance only to a percentage of people experiencing non-melancholic depression.

As yet, no formal trial has compared St John's Wort to an SSRI, but such data are expected to emerge in the next year. While the status of St John's Wort as an antidepressant remains to be clarified, its effectiveness is likely to be limited to non-melancholic depressive disorders.

St John's Wort can have side-effects, however, and there are now several reports suggesting that it may have some toxic effects on reproductive functioning. As with any drug, care should be taken to consider its side-effect profile.

How quickly do antidepressants work?

Most treatment guidelines suggest that antidepressants may take many weeks to work. It is argued that even if the current treatment seems ineffective, it should be persisted with for several weeks or even months. The Mood Disorders Unit interprets the evidence differently.

If medication is likely to be effective, evidence of at least some improvement should appear in the first ten days or so, whether it be an improvement in mood, sleep or other features. For melancholic and psychotic depression, the rate of improvement is generally slower (but relatively constant). It may, in fact, appear painfully slow.

If no improvement is noted in the first two weeks after commencing an antidepressant, the dose of that drug may need to be increased, a change to another class of antidepressant may be required, or 'augmenting' strategies (the addition of quite differing drugs) may need to be introduced. Unfortunately, when changing from one drug to another, days to weeks may pass before success can be established. It might also be the case that non-drug strategies will be more effective in bringing the depression to an end.

☆ Tranquillisers

Antidepressant drugs are significantly different from the class of drugs known as tranquillisers. This class can be divided into minor and major types.

Minor tranquillisers

Most of the minor tranquillisers belong to a family of drugs called benzodiazepines, examples of which include Ativan, Ducene, Mogadon, Murelax, Normison, Rivotril, Rohypnol, Serepax, Temazepan, Valium and Xanax.

Benzodiazepines are addictive, and may exacerbate depression, or interfere with the normal grief process. In recent years, they have been greatly overused, leading to an understandable suspicion of psychiatric medication. An unfortunate effect of this over-prescription has been a misplaced fear of antidepressants, as people don't understand that, unlike tranquillisers, they are not addictive.

Major tranquillisers

The major tranquillisers (also known as neuroleptic or antipsychotic drugs) are of particular benefit in treating psychotic depression when administered together with an antidepressant.

The newer 'atypical' antipsychotic drugs have a different side-effect profile, generally making them more tolerable to patients. As well as being effective in treating psychotic depression, they may also be of some assistance in instances of treatment-resistant melancholia. If they are effective, results are often rapid.

Antipsychotics are thought to work by blocking the action of a neurotransmitter dopamine. There are two main groups of antipsychotics—typical and atypical.

The term 'atypical' has many meanings. As a class, these drugs are serotonin–dopamine antagonists (SDAs), interacting with key brain dopamine pathways. They have different side-effects to older 'typical' antipsychotics; in particular, they are less likely to cause muscle stiffness, and appear safe and more able to be tolerated.

☆ Antimanic drugs or mood stabilisers

Bipolar disorder affects about 1–2 per cent of adults in the community, with more than 50 per cent of these people likely to experience the condition before the age of 30.

By decreasing both the frequency and amplitude of the mood swings, the antimanic medications lithium, valproate and carbamazepine (usually called mood stabilisers) are generally viewed as equally effective in the treatment of bipolar disorder. (Lithium is also used to strengthen [or augment] antidepressants when they are ineffective in dealing with unipolar depression. Such a role appears to be of likely benefit only to those with melancholic depression.) It has been suggested that each treatment may have specific advantages, depending on their different side-effects and the profile of the disorder.

Many patients who do not respond to or tolerate a particular antimanic medication will usually do well with one of the others, while patients with severe cases of bipolar disorder may require combination therapies. Particularly severe cases may require the additional use of one of the major tranquillisers.

Antimanic medications are effective in both treating episodes of mania and preventing relapses into mania and depression. When unsuccessful, combinations of mood stabilisers, or the introduction of more experimental mood stabilisers (for example, lamotrigine and topiramate) may be trialled. (These drugs are experimental in the sense that their clinical effectiveness and utility are still being clarified.)

When someone is experiencing a manic episode, all mood stabilisers generally take several weeks or more to work. For this reason, it is usually necessary to also prescribe a calming

Table 14.2   Typical and atypical antipsychotics

	Proprietary name	Generic name
Typical		
Phenothiazines	Largactil	Chlorpromazine
	Melleril	Thioridazine
	Stelazine	Trifluoperazine
	Modecate	Fluphenazine
Butyrophenones	Serenace	Haloperidol
	Droleptan	Droperidol
Diphenylbutylpiperidines	Orap	Pimozide
Thioxanthenes	Navane	Thiothixene
	Fluanxol	Flupenthixol
	Clopixol	Zuclopenthixol
Atypical	Zyprexa	Olanzapine
	Risperdal	Risperidone
	Clozaril	Clozapine
	Seroquel	Quetiapine

medication, such as a tranquilliser, which is then withdrawn once the mania settles. Someone experiencing mania often has no awareness or insight into the changes of behaviour that are occurring. The patient cannot understand the need for treatment—a need that is obvious to friends and family. Recovery takes at least several weeks, sometimes months. For someone with a first-onset episode, six months of ongoing treatment may be sufficient to prevent a relapse. The more severe or frequent the episodes, the more compelling the argument for long-term treatment.

Some people with bipolar disorder find it difficult to take the mood stabiliser regularly. This may be due to a reluctance to accept the diagnosis or the need to take medication regularly, or to see whether they can manage without tablets. Called 'poor compliance', it is a common reason for relapsing into a new episode. (In such cases, it is important to understand why the medication was stopped.) Others, however, experience further episodes despite excellent compliance.

Patients and families need to understand that most people who experience a manic episode will have further episodes of mania and/or depression.

☆ Commonly asked questions about drug treatments

Three of the most common questions asked by patients when discussing their drug treatments are:

- Must I take medication?
- How long will I need to stay on medication?
- Which drugs should I consider and what are their side-effects?

☆ Must I take medication?

There is no general rule about the need to take medication. Someone who presents with a recent non-melancholic depression that came on after a major stressor, and who has few clinical symptoms, will often do well without the need for antidepressants.

If, however, depression came on for no good reason, sleep patterns are affected, lack of emotional control is making the condition worse, or the doctor thinks the patient might have a melancholic depression, then it would be best to trial an antidepressant.

With non-melancholic depression, there is no one treatment. It's a bit like deciding what to do when a car runs off the road into a ditch. If advice to rev the engine (counselling, psychotherapy) is moving the car back towards firm ground, fine. But if all that is happening is that the wheels are spinning, it's better to put a sack under the tyres to aid grip or call a tow-truck (medication) as well. As noted on pages 75–6, many antidepressants, particularly the SSRIs, act on a patient's predisposing and perpetuating personality traits (such as

'worrying'). They may therefore indirectly prevent the onset—
as well as shorten the duration—of depressive episodes.

When deciding to stop taking an antidepressant, the patient
must check how to taper the dose. Suddenly ceasing all medication without slowly decreasing the dose can lead to severe
emotional and physical reactions including anxiety, agitation,
insomnia, severe sweats and racing heart. For some medications,
even missing one dose can initiate a 'withdrawal reaction'.

For melancholic or psychotic depression, the advantages and
need for physical treatments are distinct, with recovery quite
unlikely to occur otherwise.

☆ How long will I need to stay on the medication?

There are many treatment guidelines that pronounce strict
rules, including views that individuals should remain on medication for life if they have experienced either one severe
depressive episode or a number of episodes. Such rules are too
prescriptive and restrictive for many of those affected. However, there is an argument for extended medication treatment
if a single episode of depression

- was extremely severe;
- put the patient at considerable risk and compromised their
  functioning for an extended period; or
- was extremely difficult to treat.

In contrast, however, a patient may have had numerous depressive episodes precipitated by social factors. At some stage in
the recovery process, these social factors become irrelevant. In
such cases, it is difficult to argue that antidepressant medication should be taken for an extended period.

Decisions on how long a patient should receive medication
should therefore be made on a case-by-case basis. The prescribing clinician will need to decide what medication will be needed

to ensure 'recovery' from a particular episode, as well as whether there is a need for 'continuation' and 'maintenance' medication to prevent subsequent episodes. Large samples of data are available to help the clinician on such issues, but the very fact that the samples are based on grouped data means that they should be used just as a guide. Once a patient has recovered, the decision whether or not to alter the dose or stop the drug will depend on the individual case.

☆ Which drugs should I consider and what are their side-effects?

The decision on which drugs to take is best decided between the individual and their treating doctor.

Most drugs generate lengthy lists of possible adverse effects, even though the probability of a patient developing most of them is, at worst, slight and in most cases negligible. However, some antidepressant drugs have potentially very severe side-effects, particularly if taken in conjunction with other drugs. It is the responsibility of the treating clinician to address these issues at the individual level.

For those seeking reference material on the side-effects of drugs, drug interactions and drug safety during pregnancy and breastfeeding, two publications are recommended: *Psychotropic Drug Guidelines* and *The Maudsley Prescribing Guidelines*.

Most pharmaceutical companies provide quite detailed product information leaflets addressing side-effects and commonly raised questions about individual drugs. Bimonthly and yearly *MIMS Manuals* (Monthly Index Medical Specialty) give detailed and abbreviated information on drug side-effects and related issues.

15

Electroconvulsive Therapy and Transcranial Magnetic Stimulation

Some depressive states, especially severe psychotic depression and melancholia, may require non-medication intervention. While there are a number of candidate strategies, we consider two in this chapter.

☆ Electroconvulsive Therapy

Electroconvulsive Therapy (ECT) is a modern psychiatric treatment that is effective for a range of psychiatric disorders, not only melancholic and psychotic depression, but also manic disorders and certain types of schizophrenia.

A recent sample of patients assessed at the Mood Disorders Unit, who had recovered from severe depression, rated ECT as the most effective treatment for their illness. More than 80 per cent of patients who have undergone ECT are willing to receive the treatment again. That said, many patients are reluctant to start a course of ECT.

While the evidence indicates that ECT is a highly effective treatment for severe expressions of all depressive sub-types, its low initial acceptability by patients and its side-effects during the treatment course argue for it being used only for a limited set of depressive conditions.

Who might need or benefit from ECT?

Generally, those who haven't responded to other treatments may benefit from ECT. However, ECT is occasionally used as a first-line treatment for patients who have responded well to ECT previously, or who have the following conditions:

- severe psychotic depression;
- severe melancholic depression (where the patient is too ill to eat or drink, is unable to take antidepressant or anti-psychotic medications, or presents an immediate risk of suicide);
- life-threatening mania (with exhaustion and delirium); and
- severe post-natal depression.

How long does ECT take to work?

Most ECT is given at a frequency of three treatments a week. As for antidepressant drugs, evidence of improvement usually occurs in the first seven to ten days (during the first four treatments), but lasting improvement and episode recovery may require many more treatments, with the standard course lasting three to four weeks.

Improvement is best judged on those days when ECT is not given.

What's the procedure?

ECT involves patients being given a general anaesthetic to bring about sleep. They are given oxygen, and medication to relax their muscles. Next, electrical stimulation is applied through electrodes attached to one or both sides of the scalp. This causes a brief convulsion. The resultant activity in the nerve cells helps to release chemicals that restore normal functioning to the brain. The changes in the nerve impulses and neurotransmitters that occur are similar to those seen during antidepressant treatment.

There are two forms of treatment—unilateral and bilateral. Unilateral ECT involves placing both electrodes on the scalp over the non-dominant hemisphere. In bilateral ECT, electrodes are put on both sides of the head. Bilateral ECT is more effective and produces a more rapid response than unilateral ECT but, as it has some side-effects, unilateral ECT is the preferred treatment.

Two doctors (one trained in psychiatry, one in anaesthetics) and a number of nurses remain with the patient in the treatment suite, a specially equipped area of a hospital's psychiatry department. Treatment is usually given in the morning after the patient has fasted from midnight the night before.

Patients are linked to both an ECG (electrocardiogram) to measure electrical events in the heart, and to an EEG (electro-encephalogram) to measure brain waves; their heart rate and blood pressure are carefully monitored during the procedure. There are also 'stimulus dosing' procedures that determine and control the most appropriate level of electrical stimulation.

The patient wakes in a recovery room about twenty minutes after the end of the treatment under observation of trained staff.

How safe is ECT and what are the side-effects?

ECT is a very safe treatment, even for those with other physical problems or illnesses. There is no evidence that it harms the brain.

There are side-effects, however, and these can include headaches (relieved with paracetamol) and some confusion, which usually clears within hours. Memory for recent events, dates, names of friends and so on may not be as good for up to a week (occasionally longer) after treatment, but many patients will find that their memories are somewhat hazy anyway from the time of their illness.

ECT still attracts adverse publicity, but it is a very effective and sometimes life-saving treatment. Abrams (1992) is a useful technical reference.

☆ Transcranial Magnetic Stimulation—an alternative to ECT?

Transcranial Magnetic Stimulation (TMS) is a procedure used by neurologists, both as a treatment and as a diagnostic procedure. A coil is held tangential to the patient's head and a magnetic field created to stimulate relevant parts of the brain. Unlike ECT, there is no need for a general anaesthetic nor is a convulsion induced.

A number of studies have been completed, assessing the effectiveness of TMS when compared to ECT. One TMS study undertaken at the Mood Disorders Unit in Sydney suggested that it was unlikely to be as effective as ECT.

Considerable development work is being done on TMS, comparing bilateral and unilateral TMS and varying the relevant stimulus parameters. No clear statement about its utility is expected for a number of years. If TMS is demonstrated to be as effective as ECT, this would be a distinct advance in the treatment of many mood disorders.

For those wishing to learn more about TMS and its technical aspects, the text by George and Belmaker (2000) is recommended.

16

Cognitive Behavioural Therapy

As noted earlier, people who develop depression—particularly those who develop non-melancholic depression—often have an ongoing negative view of themselves, even when they are not depressed. They distort their experiences through a negative filter and develop thinking patterns that are so entrenched they don't even notice the errors of judgment caused by thinking irrationally.

Depressed people tend to focus on their shortcomings and ignore their positive points. They may also read rejection and criticism into events that are, in fact, neutral. If things go wrong, they may assume that it is their fault, and the future might seem packed with potential disasters for them and their families. Even pleasant things can be interpreted in negative ways, leading to feelings of distress. So, people who think in this way often enough will end up feeling low, having talked themselves into this frame of mind.

Here is an example of the cycle of *event–faulty thinking–reaction*:

- Your best friend forgets your birthday. *(Event)*
- You think, 'If she really liked and cared for me, she wouldn't have forgotten my birthday. I guess no one really cares about me. I'm worthless.' *(Faulty thinking)*
- Depression, loss of self-esteem. *(Reaction)*

Cognitive Behaviour Therapy (CBT) brings a problem-solving approach to the identification of thoughts and behaviours that precipitate and perpetuate depression.

In the sequence—*event–thought–reaction*—most people aren't consciously aware of the step in the middle: thought. Habits of mind aren't a problem unless we find ourselves constantly feeling bad. We then need to look at the way we are thinking and see whether we need to change some of our thinking habits.

CBT is aimed at making patients aware of their thinking habits and how they contribute to feelings of depression. It aims to change negative thinking habits so that people can stop themselves feeling so bad. It is also something they can learn to do for themselves.

Either in one-on-one therapy sessions or in small groups, the therapist teaches people to look logically and rationally at the evidence for their negative thinking, thus helping them adjust the way they view the world around them.

The therapist will provide 'homework' for between sessions. Patients may be asked sensitive questions such as:

- What do you think of yourself?
- What do you make of your experiences?
- How do you view the future?

This is really extended self-therapy. By using CBT tools and observing the way they think about their world, patients will find out how to examine the truth, or otherwise, of their everyday assumptions and interpretations. Thinking negatively is a habit and, like any other bad habit, it can be broken.

☆ Schemas, and learning to reframe them

The concept of schemas comes from the idea that children evaluate themselves and their environment through interaction with significant others, in order to construct their own 'reality'. Automatic thoughts and other evaluations of day-to-day experiences that tend to reinforce or support these 'realities' are known as 'underlying assumptions'.

Underlying assumptions may be adaptive and lead to positive attitudes (for example, 'I will have a go at most things and do a reasonable job' or 'People are basically helpful'). They may also be dysfunctional (for example, 'I have to be the best at everything' or 'People generally let me down') and leave a person vulnerable to the onset of depression, or at risk of subsequent relapse.

People can learn to reframe and modify their existing schema or deeply entrenched assumptions, as well as modify their approach to problem-solving and the life values they hold as a result of early experiences. There are four steps to achieving this:

Step 1: Appraise the situation leading to depression.
What is going on? What is the pattern? What are my reasons for reacting this way? Are they justified? Where is this getting me?

Step 2: Evaluate thoughts and beliefs triggered by events.
What is the evidence for how I am thinking? What would it take to make it change? How strongly do I believe in these thoughts and feelings? How much do I have invested in this?

Step 3: Substitute helpful thoughts.
How else can I view this? What is another way of looking at this? What has worked for me in the past? What would the helpful part of me advise?

Step 4: Try out new ways of thinking and behaving.
What new idea or option can I try? If, by some miracle, things were different, how would they be different? What is required to make this difference? What option will I try first?

Becoming aware of our thoughts

Whenever we feel very upset, depressed, guilty or angry, we should stop what we're doing and try to become aware of

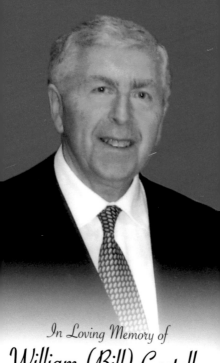

In Loving Memory of

William (Bill) Costello
Tybroughney, Piltown,
Co. Kilkenny
who died on 8th December 2014
Aged 72 years
May he rest in peace

A silent thought,
A quite prayer
For a special person
in God's care.

"May He support us

all the day long,

till the shadows lengthen,

and the evening comes,

and the busy world is hushed,

and the fever of life is over,

and our work is done !

Then in His mercy

may He give us a

safe lodging,

and a holy rest, and

peace at last."

Cardinal Newman

Raggett © T: 087 2202391 www.kilkennycards.ie

what we are thinking, or what images are going through our minds. If we find ourselves saying 'I felt that . . .' or 'I thought that . . .', we are probably about to express a thought and not a feeling. For example, 'I felt that he had no right to say that to me' is a thought, not a feeling.

We can all identify some of the familiar put-downs we use against ourselves, or the negative thoughts we have about ourselves, for example:

'I'm hopeless at . . .'
'Everyone is smarter than me.'
'I'll never get over what he said to me . . .'

The aim is to gather more accurate information about our thoughts so that we can pinpoint and counteract distortions.

Some faulty thinking habits

Let's look at a character called Bill who, unfortunately for him, illustrates all of the following faulty thinking habits.

Black and white thinking. Bill sees an event either as a success or a total failure. He evaluates everything in extremes. Take, for example, his thoughts about this week's tennis match: 'I've got to be perfect this week, I was so lousy last Sunday.'

Generalising. Bill needs only one example of behaviour to make a general rule for all times and all places. He forgets that behaviour is very much determined by a specific situation, such as the other person's mood. For example, Bill's tennis partner, Ted, is not very talkative today. (Bill doesn't know that Ted's dog died last night.) Bill thinks, 'Ted doesn't like playing tennis with me—nobody has ever really enjoyed my company.'

Getting things out of proportion. Bill focuses on an event that would be unpleasant (for anyone), but builds the situation up to an extreme. For example, Bill has made a mistake at work. He thinks, 'How incompetent of me. That's blown my chances with the boss. No-one else would have made such a stupid mistake. I'm hopeless.' He also treats criticism as total rejection.

Personalising a situation. If someone is angry or upset, Bill thinks it is his fault or his responsibility. He feels that things are happening this way because of him. For example, tennis has been rained out. Ted was looking forward to the exercise, and now he is grumpy. Bill thinks, 'Ted is mad at me because this is the second Sunday that I've booked for tennis and it's rained. I'm embarrassed—it's rained two Sundays in a row!'

Setting unrealistic expectations. Bill believes that it is essential to be perfect and in control at all times. For example, he finds taking his two-year-old, Sam, to a restaurant an irritating experience. He loses his temper with Sam because he is messy and noisy. Bill thinks, 'I should be able to control Sam better. I'm a hopeless parent, always yelling at him.'

Arbitrary inference. Bill often draws conclusions or inferences from situations where there is no evidence to support conclusions. He then uses these inferences to put himself down. For example, 'Everyone else looks happy all the time. I should be happy all the time. I'm a failure if I feel unhappy.'

Selective abstraction. Bill is sensitive, always on the lookout for signs of rejection or criticism. He dwells on things that others have said or done and interprets them as critical of himself. 'Ted rushed off straight after tennis today. I think he finds me boring. He didn't want to stop for coffee.' (Ted was, in fact, under orders to be home on time after tennis to put on the barbecue for guests.)

Learning rational thinking

Rational thinking is realistic thinking, not simply positive thinking. Sometimes 'positive' thoughts can be irrational and leave a person feeling just as down. For example, 'This time I *will* succeed. It'll be different to every other time.'

Such a self-instruction is irrational as it sets up unrealistic expectations that will only lead to feelings of failure and despair if things don't work out. Of course, we should all allow for faults, mistakes, bad moods and unpleasant feelings over the course of an ordinary day. The trick is not to let such feelings overcome us.

The way we talk to ourselves influences the way we feel and behave. For example, 'I feel upset about what just happened, but I can't do anything about it. I'll distract myself by keeping busy. I won't let myself dwell on it' instead of, 'Oh no! How can I face the rest of the day after this! I'm too upset to work. Today is a disaster'. People who continually tell themselves 'I can't cope' will end up believing it. This will prevent them from learning new ways of coping.

Here are some of the common irrational beliefs that can have a very negative effect on thought patterns.

- It is essential that people I think are important to me should like/love/approve of me all the time. If they don't, it must mean that I'm bad/worthless.
- I must be good at what I do and always try to improve myself.
- Some people are bad/wicked/evil and I should be very upset by their behaviour.
- It is a total disaster if things don't work out the way I want.
- Fate/destiny controls us. We have little to do with causing our own sorrows or unhappiness.
- If something is, or may be, dangerous or frightening, I must be concerned about it and worry about it happening to me.
- If things are too hard it's better to avoid them than fail.
- We must have others to rely on. We all need someone stronger than ourselves in order to cope with life.

- What happened in my past will always affect me—both now and in the future.
- I should be very upset and dwell on other people's problems and crises if I really care for them.

Changing the way we think, by being aware of our thoughts, involves three stages:

Anticipation—before the event.
Reaction—during the event.
Analysis—after the event.

How someone looks forward to an activity is very important in laying the groundwork for their emotional response. For example, if an invitation to a party brings an emotional response such as, 'I won't know anyone there. I'll look so stupid', then negative thinking has to be stopped before it starts. It is completely self-defeating. More self-encouraging statements would be: 'I might find the party a bit of a strain but I'll get myself a drink and stand in the kitchen. I might be able to offer some food around and get to talk to people that way.'

Self-talk in any situation will make a difference to the way someone copes. Negative thoughts after an event will make it harder to face that activity in future. Develop the habit of thinking logically rather than emotionally. For example: 'I'm shy at parties, but they are an important part of meeting people. What can I do to cope better? Which "bits" worry me most?'

Thought stopping

Thought stopping is a useful technique to interrupt negative thinking.

- Say 'STOP! STOP!' to yourself, as loudly as you can, in your head and simultaneously imagine a stop sign.

• Immediately distract yourself by concentrating on regulating your breathing, relaxing, thinking of something positive or imagining something pleasant.

Author note: The material in this chapter has been adapted from a treatment manual prepared by our clinical psychologist colleagues Susan Tanner and Jillian Ball. For further details and practical exercises, see Tanner and Ball (1999).

17

Interpersonal Therapy

Interpersonal Therapy (IPT) is also of relevance to the non-melancholic disorders. It makes no assumption about the origin of the depression, and uses the connection between onset of depressive symptoms and current interpersonal problems as a treatment focus. The underlying assumption is that depressive symptoms and interpersonal problems are interrelated.

Clinical depression is seen as having three components:

- *symptom formation*, that is, the development of depressive **affect** based on psychological and biological origins;
- *social functioning*, that is, where social interactions are derived from childhood experience, current social reinforcement and/or personal attempts at competence and mastery and of social and interpersonal situations; and
- *personality*, including the handling of guilt and anger. These enduring traits constitute a person's unique pattern of reactions and functioning, some of which can contribute to depressive symptomatology.

IPT generally deals with current rather than past interpersonal relationships and focuses on the immediate social context. It attempts to intervene in symptom formation and social dysfunction associated with depression, rather than changing enduring aspects of personality.

The onset of any depression occurs in a social or interpersonal context. IPT works on the premise that understanding the context can help the individual identify depression, master it, deal with it and prevent it recurring.

The goals in IPT are:

- to demystify depression (depression doesn't just come 'out of the blue' and it can be mastered);
- to provide strategies for dealing with depression by making a 'diagnosis' about some of the causes, by educating the individual to establish links between symptoms and feelings, by exploring the interpersonal context, and by identifying the problem areas and making them explicit; and
- to improve the individual's interpersonal functioning.

Once the problem area has been identified, the therapist can give the patient a framework explaining where therapy is going and what might be achieved. IPT doesn't aim to change personality, but it helps deal with the current stressful situation.

The four broad areas where IPT can be helpful are:

- unresolved grief (either fresh or from the past): for example, difficulty in grieving the death of a parent because of unresolved anger;
- disputes (which could be marital, with children, or at work);
- transitions: for example, when a child leaves home, when there is a change of job, separation, divorce or on retirement; and
- interpersonal shortfalls: for example, if a person lacks assertiveness, is feeling lonely or bored, or has difficulty in initiating or sustaining relationships.

☆ Techniques

While the techniques of IPT are generic to psychotherapy (that is, to listen, empathise, deal with a person's feelings and help them to talk freely about their worries and concerns), the therapy occurs in three main phases.

First, the therapist has to make a diagnostic evaluation of the patient and obtain an appropriate psychiatric history. This involves a review of symptoms, a diagnosis and an explanation of the interpersonal context for the depression. The therapist reviews the patient's current social functioning and current close relationship patterns, as well as the mutual expectations and changes involved in these relationships prior to the onset of the depression. This review provides the framework and defines the focus of treatment.

In the second phase, the therapist explores with the patient the identified interpersonal problem area, and a contract for treatment is discussed. The contract should outline the likely number of sessions the patient will need and the therapeutic goals, as well as touch on what each party might expect of the other.

The final phase of therapy encourages the patient to recognise and consolidate what has been learnt, as well as develop ways of identifying and countering depressive symptoms in the future.

A standard course usually involves 12–16 sessions. A useful reference on IPT is Weissman (1995).

Session Therapy Outline

---

1. An explanation of IPT and an assessment of the patient's background and details. The therapist will elicit information using an interpersonal inventory.
2. The contract. The therapist makes explicit what the therapy hopes to achieve and the length of time the therapy is expected to last.
3. An exploration of past and present relationships in order to explore the facets of the patient's personality that led to the current difficulties.
4. A closer exploration of interpersonal incidents with questions asked such as, how did this particular situation occur? The emphasis is on what this exploration reveals to the patient about himself/herself.
5. A discussion of other behaviours possible in response to the situation.
6. An exploration of important incidents in and around the current situation and what the legitimate expectations might be.

7. An exploration of decision making. Working out future directions and expectations for the future.
8. Assignment of 'homework' that will help to clarify the problem.
9. Feedback to the therapist about the outcome of the homework.
10. Closure. A discussion with the patient about what has been learnt.

18

Psychotherapies and counselling

There are many 'types' of psychotherapy and counselling, all with varying emphases and approaches. Each may be useful in specific situations.

Psychotherapy

By definition, psychotherapy comprises a working relationship between a trained therapist and a patient. Psychotherapy emerged from psychoanalytic techniques that included encouraging patients to 'free associate'. The therapist would then progressively clarify and interpret links between the past and the present.

'Brief' psychodynamic psychotherapy seeks to overcome the intensive and extended nature of psychoanalysis. While this form of psychotherapy might involve exploring issues such as 'transference' (feelings about significant others in the past being projected onto the therapist), it seeks to focus on a particular problem, such as depression. Goals might be to explore how an individual developed depression (perhaps, by pursuing aspects of current relationships) or developed a propensity to depression (by considering aspects of the patient's background such as low self-worth as a consequence of harsh and punitive parenting, or childhood abuse). The direct aim of brief psychotherapy is to assist the development of insight. However, the non-judgmental support offered by psychotherapy can also be of distinct help to many depressed individuals.

When this is the principal aim, the approach may be called 'supportive psychotherapy'.

There are limitations to the brief psychotherapies. Treatment may, in fact, not be brief, but often extend for months and sometimes years. There may be a lack of structure, so that even after months in therapy the patient may be quite unclear about the goals and objectives. 'Dependency' on the therapist can also develop. While this may be appropriate on a short-term basis, if it is not resolved or 'worked through' the individual's intrinsic capacity to deal (or not deal) with situations and thus build up a level of resilience may be taken away. The capacity for therapy to drift when applied by less skilled therapists has led to the development of quite structured psychotherapies, with Cognitive Behavioural Therapy and Interpersonal Therapy being perhaps the best examples (see Chapters 16 and 17).

Effective therapists tend to be empathic (good listeners), non-judgmental (trained to listen without being critical), and do not dictate what people should do. Their attitude, which is often one of unconditional positive regard for the patient, should encourage patients to 'ventilate' (talk about things that are concerning and preoccupying them).

Therapists may use the trusting and accepting relationship that should grow between them and the patient (the therapeutic relationship) as a microcosm (a smaller, safer version of the outside world) to understand how the patient acts in everyday life. Therapy may be structured to a particular pattern or follow the priorities set by either party.

As there are so many types of psychotherapy, effectiveness depends on the skill of the therapist and the readiness and ability of the patient to embark on such a venture. Psychotherapy may be particularly helpful for those with non-melancholic depression, but it is not a first-line treatment for melancholic or psychotic depression.

☆ Counselling

There are many techniques and applications for counselling. These are generally most useful when patients are either stressed or in crisis as it is at this time that they are most amenable to changing set behaviours.

Much counselling focuses on problem solving. The counsellor may, therefore, be of particular help in listening to a wide range of issues, clarifying and ranking key problems, identifying those that may require or benefit from action, encouraging the individual to act and then considering the results of such actions. Marital counselling and career advice are examples of the type of problem solving a counsellor may undertake. Career advice identifies an important aspect of counselling—the provision of practical well-informed help.

Crisis counselling may also involve problem solving but will also seek ways to reduce an individual's stress levels. This can involve strategies to relieve any potential or actual post-traumatic stress reaction. While self-help is encouraged, the counsellor may also provide practical help.

Counsellors may range from those who are very directive to those who encourage patients to determine their own options. Such contrasting styles have their own predictable advantages and disadvantages. Whatever approach is taken, a counsellor should interact in a way that inspires trust and confidence.

19

Anger management

In writing about her depression, the broadcaster Helen Razor introduced the concept of Van Pelt's Disorder. Named after Lucy Van Pelt in the Peanuts cartoon strip, this disorder invokes an image of someone 'snatching their paltry little Linus blankets and tripping over them relentlessly and kicking them in their adipose Charlie Brown arses'.[1]

Anger is clearly a powerful and complex emotion. It can be tangled up with depression and is difficult to deal with effectively. Anger can arise from situations or life experiences that have caused disappointment, hurt or fright. It can also be in response to a violation of physical or psychological 'territory'. Individual physiological as well as psychological differences mean that some people get angrier than others, and some find it harder to control their temper than others. Those who are 'placid' by temperament have less of a problem, but the rest of us have to deal with uncomfortable levels of anger from time to time.

Most people find anger difficult to manage, but we can learn to use the energy that anger provides in constructive ways, rather than 'bottling it up', 'stewing', turning the anger inwards ('acting in'), being hostile, volatile or irritable, or 'exploding' ('acting out').

Cognitive Behavioural Therapy (CBT) can be of distinct use for those with an internalising personality style. It may also be very helpful to those with an externalising personality style, that is, where the individual is irritable and reports 'biting people's heads off'. However, there are some additional or alternative strategies worth highlighting here. These are:

- recognise that you are angry;
- identify what made you angry;
- establish what you can do about these feelings of anger; and
- release your anger in alternative ways.

☆ Recognise that you are angry

Many people don't recognise anger. Their feelings come out as 'hurt' or 'fear'. They feel powerless, belittled or humiliated and don't want to dwell on these feelings. Others ruminate on the experiences that have made them angry and nourish grudges. Some become sour, vindictive or depressed.

It is common to fear anger's destructive force. In many families, therefore, displays of anger are not tolerated: they may be stifled in the children, and repressed in parents. This can happen regardless of whether or not the anger is justified, leading to an added level of confusion and discomfort for those who are feeling angry. There is generally a 'taboo' on expressing anger, or even feeling it.

We should consider our own behaviour. Are we being deliberately provocative or irritable? Perhaps passive aggressive? It may be that the person who is making us angry reminds us of the less attractive parts of our own character. If we recognise *why* we are angry, this can help us to control the anger.

Don't shy away from anger, acknowledge it.

☆ Identify what made you angry

Anger is a signal that all is not well. We should give shape to our feelings as to do so judiciously is neither bad nor childish, but mature. We should identify the situations that make us particularly angry. Are we being overlooked or taken for granted? Have we had to compromise something we believe in? Has someone taken or violated something precious to us or to someone we value?

Once we have cooled off a little, we should ask, is our anger 'reasonable'? Is it in proportion to the situation that caused it? An intense reaction probably reflects that the immediate cause of the anger has triggered off energy from older, unresolved hurts and fears—perhaps from as far back as childhood.

☆ Establish what we can do about these feelings of anger

We can use our understanding of what gave rise to our anger to learn about ourselves. There are certain actions we can take that will ameliorate our feelings somewhat. Try and work out what these are and ask a (disinterested) friend what they think. Sometimes past hurts, injustices or indignities can be resolved with those responsible. If this is not possible, a skilled therapist can help heal the bruises. Sometimes we can forgive, or at least move on. Situations or conflicts that are unresolvable should be avoided. It is difficult to change others' attitudes, but we can improve our own. Each of us has control over ourselves.

☆ Release your anger in alternative ways

Expressing anger can be tricky, which is why it is better to be at some distance from the raw emotion. So, don't 'see red', don't 'let it all out', instead 'cool it' and get back to the rational self. Go for a brisk walk, beat up a cushion, or scream long and loud while face down in a pillow. Alternatively, write a 'bottom drawer' letter expressing exactly what you would say if the situation occurred all over again. (Just *don't post* it). Read it the next day, laugh at it and get your course of action more judiciously worked out. You will eventually calm down and therefore be better equipped to make decisions about what to do.

This doesn't mean, however, that we should not express our anger, just that it is often wise not to do so in the heat of the moment. We are often pretty inarticulate when indignant, so attempting to communicate while very angry will probably be counterproductive.

Communication with the person who caused the feelings of anger will only help if we can express clearly what has angered us, and what we see as the solution to the problem. Try to be direct: sarcasm, scorn, casting blame or character analysis will only make a messy situation messier. We may even be able to listen to the other person's point of view. We are not responsible for their feelings, so should try to find this approach unthreatening.

There may be a compromise that suits all parties, and this is far better than maintaining a 'cold war' of silences and passive aggression, which is wearing for everyone involved, solves nothing and can turn us into 'victims'. Things don't change overnight, however, and we sometimes have to state our point of view firmly and objectively, more than once, and 'stick to our guns'.

Sometimes we are unable to state our anger because the person or situation that provoked it is 'out of reach'. This may be because of a professional relationship (boss/employee), illness, a closeness where frankness may be a risk, or where intimacy is not desired. In each case there are solutions although it may take a chat with a friend or a therapist to find them. However, such chats should never be used simply to reiterate your original anger.

Some solutions could take a lot of courage. For example, if you are continually angry with your boss, consider that you have genuine cause for such feelings and that it is not just unrealistic expectations on your part, then the only solution may be to change jobs.

Finally, what about that unexpressed slow-burning anger, resentment? Resentment may arise from a feeling of being exploited. For example, in today's busy marriages, a partner can feel worn out from time to time, and resent that the other seems not to be pulling their weight. While this may not necessarily be the case, in such a situation both partners need to be direct with one another and seek creative solutions to the problem so that each gets a little spare time. Go somewhere quiet and try to nut out a solution. If the situation cannot be changed, strategies will have to be developed so that resentment doesn't rule you.

In the earlier chapters, it was noted that a significant percentage of those with non-melancholic depression feel more irritable and angry with others when depressed. These are, in fact, the commonest expressions of non-melancholic depression in young people. Although they overlap, irritability and anger often have differing origins.

Irritability is best viewed as the externalised expression of anxiety. It is thus likely to be episodic, expressed when an individual is stressed or depressed, and often to their later embarrassment. ('I'm really embarrassed at how I've been behaving recently—biting my partner's head off and criticising the children, when they haven't really done anything wrong.') The expression of irritability during a non-melancholic depressive episode therefore favours anxiety management before an anger management program.

By contrast, those who get angry tend to have a more ongoing volatile personality style, and are less tolerant of and more frustrated by stressors. They reduce stress by blaming others rather than themselves and are less likely to be embarrassed at involving others in their 'hissy fits'. If the person is motivated, an anger management program is generally one of the best initial strategies.

20

Matching the treatment to the depression

I cannot imagine leading a normal life without both taking lithium and having had the benefits of psychotherapy . . . lithium . . . diminishes my depressions . . . gentles me out . . . But, ineffably, psychotherapy heals.

Kay Jamison, *An Unquiet Mind*

As noted in the Introduction, depression is commonly viewed as an 'it', as if there is just one condition that varies dimensionally—whether by severity, persistence or recurrence. Defining 'depression' in such a way (with official systems listing 'major' and 'minor' depression as if such distinctions are illuminating) has consolidated the 'it' model. Acceptance of this 'non-specificity' model has had two principal results. The first is that patients are likely to receive a treatment favoured by their practitioner rather than a therapy tailored to their condition on a demonstrated and rational basis. There is a 'one size fits all' model for viewing the treatments for the depressive disorders. As evaluative studies have shown a similar response rate for non-melancholic depression across most therapies tested (whether antidepressant drugs, Cognitive Behavioural Therapy or counselling), the 'non-specificity' model has been allowed to grow unchallenged. As the psychiatrist John Ellard has observed, classifying by severity and not by cause, and then randomly assigning people to a treatment, is as rational as randomly allocating people in pain 'to spend a month in a pain program or to have an appendectomy'.

The second result of the 'non-specificity' model allows treatment to be prioritised along disciplinary lines. Doctors may model 'depression' as a disease and therefore treat patients with only antidepressant drugs. Cognitive psychologists, on the other hand, may view Cognitive Behavioural Therapy as the only appropriate treatment for 'it'.

It has been argued here that there are multiple expressions of 'depression'. In a sense, depression is a signal like pain. The diagnosis of pain is not as important as diagnosing the cause of the pain, for then treatment becomes more rational and predictable. To prescribe an analgesic for pain may be helpful (and, at times, sufficient), but it may also be less important than determining what is causing the pain and addressing that cause.

Similarly, it is important to distinguish the three principal classes of depression—psychotic, melancholic and non-melancholic. Such classifications reject the 'non-specificity' model, with psychotic and melancholic depression responding to quite differing treatment approaches. Recommendations for managing the non-melancholic disorders are less clear as it is not a pure class and, as noted, published studies suggest rather similar levels of success across quite sharply contrasting treatment approaches. This unsatisfactory finding reflects conceptualisation and measurement according to a dimensional model (of mood severity, persistence and recurrence), rather than acknowledging that non-melancholic depression may better be seen as a reflection of the painful impact between life stress and the individual's personality or temperament. The management of non-melancholic depression might therefore be advanced by developing a specific model that identifies and favours certain treatments above others for each of the major personality dimensions. Such a model might suggest antidepressant medication as being more beneficial for certain temperaments (say those with 'anxious worrying styles') than Cognitive Behavioural Therapy, and deliver the converse finding for those with a 'self-blaming' temperament style.

However, until depressive disorders are conceptualised with some specificity, such a model cannot be developed beyond a set of suggestions as set out in Table 20.1. Here, reasonably firm data for identifying the comparative benefits of differing treatments for psychotic and melancholic depression have been detailed. For the non-melancholic depressive disorders, however, it would be unwise to proceed beyond considering recommendations based on subdividing personality and temperament into 'internalising' and 'externalising' types. Table 20.1 does, however, provide a model for conceding that one particular treatment may be highly effective for one type of depression and completely ineffective for another.

Research at the Mood Disorders Unit seeks to develop a richer framework in the future. This would allow depressed individuals to receive treatment recommendations based on the 'cause' of their depression (be it biological, psychological or social) and a probability estimate of their likely response to quite contrasting treatments. This is what patients expect for their general medical problems. It is regrettable that such a situation does not currently hold for the management of depression.

The details in Table 20.1 will now be briefly outlined.

☆ Non-melancholic clinical depression

For non-melancholic clinical depression, there is a significant chance (say 20–40 per cent) that the depressive episode will remit spontaneously. That chance is increased by another 10–20 per cent if the individual receives:

• appropriate professional assessment;
• a comprehensive and clear formulation; and
• basic counselling strategies for handling the episode and its consequences.

The relatively high response rate will be lifted further

Table 20.1   **Treatment options for depression**

	Non-melancholic depression		Melancholic depression	Psychotic depression
	Internalising type	Externalising type		
Medication				
Antipsychotic (AP)	Not recommended	Not recommended	Rarely needed, but an ' 'atypical' may be very effective as an adjunct	Usually needed in conjunction with an antidepressant and highly effective
Antidepressants:				
TCA or Irreversible MAOI	Sometimes effective	Sometimes effective	Highly effective	Generally effective with an AP, rarely effective alone
SSRIs	Very effective	Sometimes very effective	Moderately effective	Commonly effective together with an AP, unlikely to be effective alone
Other 'newer' anti-depressants	Effectiveness still being investigated*	Effectiveness still being investigated*	Effectiveness still being investigated*	Effectiveness still being investigated*
Other treatments				
ECT	Not recommended	Not recommended	Effective—but rarely needed	Highly effective—but needed only by a minority
Psychotherapy (including CBT and IPT)	May be useful and effective	Useful and often effective	Of help in addition to other treatment	Of help in addition to other treatment
Counselling	Needed alongside any other treatment	Needed alongside any other treatment	Needed alongside any other treatment	Needed alongside any other treatment

* 'Effectiveness still being investigated' refers to whether these antidepressants are any more, or less, effective than the SSRIs. Combination serotonergic and noradrenergic drugs (e.g. venlafaxine, mirtazapine) may be more effective overall than the SSRIs for melancholic depression.

(perhaps by an additional 10–30 per cent) with specific treatments for the depression, which could involve:

- a course of an antidepressant drug;
- psychotherapy; or
- a combination of both.

An SSRI drug would be the most commonly anticipated first-line antidepressant prescribed, both because of its efficacy rate and because it may modify some 'drivers' of the episode (for example, anxiety, irritability, anxious worrying).

A course of psychotherapy might also have a direct antidepressant effect, either by providing the patient with strategies for addressing the episode's causes or through the support of the therapist. Psychotherapy can also address episode 'drivers', such as faulty thinking patterns.

A combination of drug treatment and psychotherapy (either commencing together or, as is more common, with psycotherapy beginning after initial drug treatment) appears to offer better results than either treatment on its own.

If one SSRI fails because of unacceptable side-effects, it may be appropriate to trial another SSRI or another antidepressant drug type. If two antidepressant drug types have been trialled at adequate dose and both have failed, then it is best to have the situation reviewed by a depression specialist. This is preferable to the traditional approach of a doctor trialling numerous antidepressants sequentially and in combination. This review might involve an assessment of the patient's primary physical condition (for example, medical conditions and medication taken), but would particularly focus on the identification and treatment of predisposing variables (for example, personality style) and depression maintenance factors, such as a dysfunctional marriage or problems with parents. As noted earlier, the individual is likely to benefit if the treatment approach addresses any predisposition emerging from personality or temperament.

☆ Melancholic depression

For melancholic depression, the chance of a spontaneous remission—with or without a professional assessment—is slight (perhaps 5–10 per cent). A physical treatment is almost always required immediately. If the patient has had previous episodes and has always responded to a particular antidepressant medication then, subject to the acceptability of any side-effects, it might be expected that the same antidepressant would be recommenced. If, however, the side-effects profile compromised treatment, it would be wise to consider introducing an alternative antidepressant.

If the episode is the patient's first, then it would be reasonable to trial an SSRI initially. If an SSRI was commenced and failed to be effective, a move to an SNRI would be the second option. At least 50 per cent of first-episode patients would be expected to respond to such a treatment, showing some evidence of improvement in the first one to three weeks.

If there is no evidence of any improvement over three weeks, it may be wise to move to another drug class rather than accept the oft-put claim that an antidepressant must be trialled for up to eight weeks. Other drug classes might include a tricyclic or an irreversible MAOI (where a higher effectiveness would be anticipated, but with certain worrying side-effects and some management difficulties) or, rarely, one of the newer classes of antidepressant (these usually have fewer side-effects, but the drugs are less effective).

If there is no evidence of improvement after trialling two or three antidepressant drugs, **augmentation** strategies (such as introducing lithium or a thyroid hormone) may be of benefit. Sometimes, an atypical antipsychotic drug might be trialled as an adjunctive drug if the patient has failed to respond to several antidepressants. If such a drug is to be effective, its benefits will be evident in a few days, and the dose should then be reduced rapidly.

If a patient has had previous episodes and received anti-depressants, it is vital for the practitioner to review the individual effectiveness of these drugs before deciding on whether to follow the above strategy or design an alternative procedure.

ECT is highly effective. This treatment should be considered if a patient has failed to experience any improvement after trialling several antidepressant drugs, or is at grave medical risk (for example, from poor nutrition or dehydration), highly suicidal and unable to be readily protected. Patients who have previously had ECT may request ECT instead of drug treatment.

In some cases where a patient has been maintained on an antidepressant drug over a period of time, the drug can become increasingly ineffective. American psychiatrists have termed this a 'poop out' effect. It may reflect stressful life events overriding the beneficial medication (which argues for an increased dose) or a true loss of effectiveness (which argues for an increased dose or a transfer to a new drug type, alone or in combination).

Non-physical treatments such as counselling or psychotherapy are best viewed as adjunctive. They may focus on physical treatment issues (for example, drug compliance, side-effects and the stigma of illness) or address issues in a patient's life that may either be linked to the depression or quite independent of it. Non-physical treatments on their own are ineffective against melancholia.

If progress is less than satisfactory after two or three treatments have been trialled, assessment by a depression specialist should occur.

☆ Psychotic depression

For psychotic depression, the spontaneous remission rate is negligible (less than 5 per cent). The two most effective treatments (with an effectiveness rate of about 80 per cent) are a combination of an antipsychotic drug and an antidepressant drug, or ECT (with bilateral ECT being slightly more effective than unilateral ECT). In most cases, it is advisable to start with drug treatment, but ECT could well be considered initially for patients who have previously been treated with ECT or who are at grave medical risk, or are highly suicidal. For those with severe agitation, a sedative medication such as a benzodiazepine can be extremely helpful.

As for melancholic depression, non-physical treatments are important adjunctives but, by themselves, are ineffective and inappropriate.

If progress is unsatisfactory, assessment by a depression specialist should occur.

☆ A note on counselling and psychotherapy

While counselling and psychotherapy have been recommended in the preceding sections, their usefulness and importance depends to a great extent on the skills and interpersonal style of the practitioner. Their potential to help should not be minimised, however. While a wide range of strategies are available (these are not easily summarised here), a good practitioner will set goals, keep the patient informed about expectations and working hypotheses, and move comfortably from addressing problems in the past to trying to prevent such problems in the future. Practitioners with good interpersonal skills will make a patient feel understood, cared about and supported, but not overly controlled or dominated. These matters of style are vitally important, yet it is difficult to define them accurately. Kay Jamison explains:

> The debt I owe my psychiatrist is beyond description
> . . . It was all the stupid, desperately optimistic, con-
> descending things he didn't say that kept me alive . . .
> all the compassion and warmth I felt from him that
> could not have been said . . . and his granite belief that

mine was a life worth saving . . . Most difficult to put into words, but in many ways the essence of everything.[1]

☆ Treatment-resistant patients

At the Mood Disorders Unit we are most commonly asked to assess patients with 'treatment resistance'. This term is used to describe the situation when a depressed patient has failed to show either an adequate response or a maintained response after receiving at least two quite different antidepressant drugs or treatments. Patients most likely to become resistant are:

- those with a non-melancholic depression whose treatment has been excessively 'biological' with numerous drugs being trialled and without enough attention being paid to issues that need to be 'talked through';
- those with melancholic depression who have been trialled on 'new' antidepressants only; and
- those who do not have a primary depressive disorder, but, instead, an anxiety condition, a medical problem, personality difficulties or substance dependence as their primary condition.

Situations such as these emphasise the importance of diagnosing depression accurately and specifying its sub-type. By clarifying the 'true' diagnosis and making treatment more rational, or by prescribing augmenting and combination treatments, most patients with treatment-resistant depression receive benefit.

21

Living with someone with depression

People seem to be able to bear or tolerate depression as long as there is the belief that things will improve.

Kay Jamison, *Night Falls Fast*

Depression and hopelessness are 'infectious' and can bring out the worst—and the best—in families. Families can slip into ways of behaving that are meant to protect the depressed person, but which, in fact, lead to overprotection and to feelings of resentment in other family members. Family members, carers, friends and the general practitioner can all become frustrated.

It is important to establish clear and effective communication within the family. This may require the whole family meeting with a professional for a few sessions. A depressive episode may provide an opportunity for family members to re-evaluate what is important in their relationships and to try to resolve 'unfinished business' such as grief, relationship difficulties, dormant regrets or guilt.

The first few weeks of treatment are often crucial. This is a time for patience, care and encouragement. The patient may not have wanted to see the psychiatrist in the first place. During the early stages of treatment, it is very common for the patient to want to give up—the drugs can throw up side-effects without providing any obvious benefits. While patients may be told that their condition *is* treatable, their depression often leads them to forget or dismiss this message. Family members should reinforce it.

It does not help to suggest that the depressed person should 'pull up their socks'. Unfortunately, this common response from family and friends can only be counterproductive, as it reinforces feelings of depression and guilt. If the depressed person is suicidal, it is important that risks be reduced and that 'protective' (but not overprotective) support systems be set up.

Family members should never suggest that drug treatment be discontinued once a particular episode is over: that is up to the individual to discuss with the treating doctor.

It is important to realise that psychotherapy can have treatment-related effects. It can put all sorts of demands on the rest of the family. It is not uncommon for depressed people to 'bottle up' their feelings, especially anger. As therapy helps them unblock some of these old feelings, there can be emotional scenes. It may appear that the patient is attacking family members, but it is important that they do not take it too personally. If there is some validity to the complaints, family members should respond appropriately. If the real issues belong further back in childhood, let the patient blow off steam. The family should stick around to be understanding as the storm abates.

Counterattacking is not helpful. Family members who feel uneasy about what therapy is doing to the patient should ask to be included in a session with the patient and the therapist. In some cases, the spotlight may be on relationships and family members may find themselves being invited into therapy sessions anyway.

Partners may be asked to resurrect 'fun' in the depressed person's life. It is at this stage that families can talk openly about the effects of living with somebody suffering depression. This can be seen as the start of a relationship resuming a more equal pattern rather than maintaining the 'carer/patient' roles that are common in the early days of depression.

It is important for all those involved in the management of depression to take steps to prevent any **recurrence**. Depressed people and their families need to recognise early warning signs and act quickly. Attention should also be paid to lifestyle changes including diet, exercise, social life and interests.

☆ Suicide

Depressive disorders can be associated with the feeling that life isn't worth living any more. Predicting just who is at risk is difficult, but statistics can give a general indication of the higher risk groups.

Psychotic depression poses a serious risk, as do symptoms of severe anxiety and agitation, or any serious physical illness. Being single, divorced, widowed, unemployed, or having a substance abuse habit increases risk. Those who have already attempted suicide are more likely to try it again.

Some warning signs are:

- repeated expressions of hopelessness or desperation;
- out-of-character behaviours, such as recklessness in a normally careful person;
- an abrupt mood change to an uncharacteristic calmness (a suicide plan may offer relief and lift mood);
- giving away prized possessions to relatives and friends;
- making out a will or taking out insurance;
- making remarks about death, dying and suicide.

Families can help by removing potentially harmful items such as tablets and firearms, and by seeking treatment as a matter of urgency. Local mental health services have 24-hour freecall helplines to provide advice and assistance. Information on child and adolescent mental health services is available from local area health services. If in doubt, ring the nearest hospital or the emergency services. If family members are concerned that the treatment plan is not addressing the patient's needs, they should ask their general practitioner for assistance or contact other community resources (see 'References and further resources' on pages 134–40). It may be difficult to obtain appropriate help—but persist.

☆ Are there any prizes?

One of the things that makes psychiatry a rewarding profession is that, not only do most depressed patients get back to their 'old selves', but it is quite common for them to learn from the experience:

> Mysterious in its coming, mysterious in its going, the affliction runs its course, and one finds peace[1].

William Styron noted that being 'restored to the capacity for serenity and joy . . . may be indemnity enough for having endured the despair beyond despair'.[2] Margo Orum indicated that in 'the end, I opted for building more meaning into my everyday life, by doing the things I love, so that now my everyday life is . . . precious . . . the pay-offs are worth it'.[3] Penelope Rowe could say 'I can "thank" my illness for shaving off some prickly edges and giving me greater tolerance (although I wish there had been an easier way!)'.[4]

In fact, some people who have dealt with depression end up emotionally stronger than they ever were before. Strategies developed to manage depression can assist the management of general life situations. This optimistic thought should be kept in mind. For some depressed people and their families, it can be a long and hard road to recovery. There is, however, a signpost at the beginning that is worth reading:

> For most people, depression is totally treatable. The endpoint is recovery, not merely improvement.

Appendix

Mood disorders, the artistic temperament and worldly 'success'

In her book *Touched with Fire*, Kay Jamison provides a lengthy list of writers, musicians and artists who have had either a depressive or bipolar disorder. They include Hans Christian Andersen, Charles Dickens, F. Scott Fitzgerald, Leo Tolstoy, Graham Greene, William Blake, Robert Burns, Lord Byron, Adam Lindsay Gordon, Emily Dickinson, Sylvia Plath, Irving Berlin, George Handel, Noel Coward, Cole Porter, Paul Gauguin, Michelangelo and Georgia O'Keefe. While her focus is on the reasons for the link between creativity and mood disorders, Kay Jamison's list also speaks to the reality that people with mood disorders can achieve and succeed in the most competitive and demanding careers when not restricted or disabled by their condition. As depression becomes less stigmatised we can expect more and more 'successful' people, be they professionals, business people or politicians, to discuss and identify how they have dealt with their mood disorder. As a psychiatrist and author of the most respected and informative book on manic-depressive illness, Kay Jamison's description of her own bipolar disorder in *An Unquiet Mind* serves as an inspiration.

Notes

Introduction

1. Wolpert, L. *Malignant Sadness.*

Chapter 2 Depression, a common experience

2. Nesse, R.M. 'Is depression an adaptation?'
3. Milligan, S. and Clare, A. *Depression and How to Survive It,* p. 41.
4. Jamison, K. *An Unquiet Mind,* pp. 218–19.

Chapter 6 General features of depression and bipolar disorders

5. Styron, W. *Darkness Visible,* p. 56.
6. Milligan, S. and Clare, A. *Depression and How to Survive It,* p. 13.
7. ibid., p. 15.
8. Jamison, K. *An Unquiet Mind,* p. 45.
9. Styron, W. *Darkness Visible,* p. 45.
10. Razor, H. *Gas Smells Awful,* pp. 132–3.
11. ibid., p. 130.
12. Jamison, K. *An Unquiet Mind,* pp. 36–7.

Chapter 9   Personality styles and non-melancholic depression

13. Jamison, K. *Night Falls Fast*, p. 197.
14. ibid., p 198.

Chapter 14   Drug treatments

1. Williams et al. *Annals of Internal Medicine.*

Chapter 19   Anger management

1. Razor, H. *Gas Smells Awful*, p. 69.

Chapter 20   Matching the treatment to the depression

1. Jamison, K. *Night Falls Fast*

Chapter 21   Living with someone with depression

1. Styron, W. *Darkness Visible*, p. 73.
2. ibid., p. 84.
3. Orum, M. 'Van Gogh and lithium'.
4. Rowe, P. 'Van Gogh and lithium'.

Glossary

Adjunctive treatment   A treatment administered alongside another treatment. This can be for an effect independent of the original treatment but is more designed to strengthen the effect of another treatment.

Affect   An individual's mood state as observed by others (for example, 'his affect was one of sadness').

Affective disorder   The group of psychiatric disorders (including both manic and depressive disorders) where an affective or mood disturbance is primary. 'Primary' indicates that this is the first-ranking condition and contributes the greatest symptom distress.

Anhedonia   A lack of pleasure. A common symptom experienced by depressed people. Anticipatory anhedonia refers to an inability to look forward to a normally pleasurable activity; consummatory anhedonia is a lack of pleasure after engaging in any such activity.

Antimanic   Medication supplied to prevent or to help stabilise the highs of bipolar disorder.

Antipsychotic   Medication provided to prevent or ameliorate a psychotic episode.

Atypical depression   A possible sub-type of depression where the symptom pattern is in contrast with the usual depression profile (for example, appetite increase rather than loss, hypersomnia rather than insomnia) and where the individual is likely to have a predisposing personality style of 'interpersonal hypersensitivity' (that is, expecting that others will not like or approve of them). Alternatively, it may be an expression of depression in those with high anxiety. Atypical depression is held to be more likely to respond positively to MAOI (monoamine oxidase inhibitor) antidepressant drugs, but is now known to respond equally well to SSRIs and CBT.

Augmentation   Where the aim is to increase the effectiveness of one medication by the addition of another.

Basal ganglia   Brain centres controlling and refining motor performance.

Bipolar depression   An episode of depression in an individual with bipolar disorder. It is almost invariably 'melancholic' in its expression.

Bipolar disorder   Where the individual has episodes of mania (or hypomania) alone or with depressive episodes at other times.

Bipolar I disorder   Where the individual has experienced episode(s) of mania, with or without a history of depressive episodes.

Bipolar II disorder   Where the individual has experienced episodes of both hypomania and depression (and has never experienced an episode of mania).

Cognition   The process of thinking. Cognitions refer to thoughts, understanding and reasoning.

Cognitive limitations   Where the individual's capacity to think or reason is impaired for some reason (for example, in severe depression or dementia).

Cognitive style   The characteristics of an individual's habits of thought, how they organise their thoughts, what intentions they attribute to others and how they communicate with them.

Combination therapy   A term used to describe two or more therapeutic agents for two or more differing symptoms (for example, an antipsychotic drug plus an antidepressant drug for psychotic features and for depression in psychotic depression).

Compliance   This is where the patient follows the therapy suggested, be it by finishing a prescribed course of medication, or otherwise being involved with a course of therapy.

Continuation therapy   A term used to describe those therapies (usually drug treatments) that are implemented after management of the acute phase of an episode. These are designed to control the last stages of the current episode and, in contrast to maintenance therapies, which refer to the next phase, and where the objective is to prevent new episodes.

Cyclothymia   Probably better used to describe a temperament style where the individual has mood swings that are part of their personality, ranging from very sociable and talkative to quiet and solitary (thus a 'cyclothymic personality'). In recent years, this term has been more used to define a sub-type and milder expression of bipolar disorder, and is categorised this way in several official classificatory systems.

Delusional depression   Where the depressed individual experiences delusions (or false beliefs) during a depressive episode, and/or hallucinations or false percepts (whether of sight, sound or other senses such as taste and smell). It is termed psychotic depression in this book. Its status remains unclear, being either a sub-type of melancholic depression or a sub-type of its own.

Depressogenic   A stressful life event that is likely to cause depression in a vulnerable individual (for example, loss of job, serious family dispute).

Distal stressors   Stressful situations that occurred many years before the onset of depression but which have disposed the individual to depressive episodes.

Diurnal variation   Where the depressed individual describes a change in mood and energy at certain times of the day. Classically, those with melancholic depression report improvements in mood and energy later in the day, those with non-melancholic depression describe the opposite, and those with psychotic depression report no diurnal variation—the depression remaining persistent and unrelieved throughout the day. Such differences are, however, not entirely specific to the differing depressive sub-types.

Dopamine   A catecholamine neurotransmitter.

Double depression   Describes episodes of acute and more severe depression (major depression) superimposed on chronic depression (dysthymia).

Drug classes   Refers to different 'families' of drugs; that is, drugs derived from different chemical backgrounds.

Drug trial   Refers to when a particular drug is tried out to test its effectiveness, which will depend on the individual patient, their particular type of depression and the acceptability of any side-effects. If the drug is not effective, then it is possible to combine or augment it with another drug, change to another drug in the same class or family, or change to a drug from another family/class.

DSM (Diagnostic and Statistical Manual)   The official diagnostic classificatory system of the American Psychiatric Association. This classifies depressive disorders largely on a dimensional basis but with secondary assignment (for those who meet criteria for major depression) to melancholic and psychotic depressive classes.

Dysthymia   A diagnosis introduced into recent North American DSMs to describe non-psychotic, non-melancholic depression that is of 'minor' severity but present for two years or more.

Endogenous depression   An old term to describe melancholic depression, to reflect the view that such a depression was not related to stress and came more from within the individual. While those with melancholic depression are somewhat less likely to report antecedent life event stressors (and their depression is commonly out of proportion to any such stressor), the lack of specificity of 'stress' to depressive sub-types argues for rejecting this term.

Episode   A 'bout' of depression. To qualify as 'clinical' depression, the episode should be present for most of the time and for two weeks or more.

Externalising personality   A style of dealing with stress by reflecting its impact behaviourally (for example, raising one's voice, driving recklessly).

Euthymia   A 'normal' mood state, neither depressed nor manic.

High   This term refers to the abnormal upswing in mood that is characteristic of hypomania or mania.

Hypersomnia   Excessive sleeping (the opposite of insomnia). This may occur in melancholic, non-melancholic and atypical depression.

Hypomania   A high that is less severe than a manic episode and without any psychotic features such as misinterpretation of events.

ICD-10   The current official International Classification of Diseases prepared by the World Health Organization. This system categorises depressive disorders principally on the basis of severity.

Improvement   When the clinical condition is somewhat better but not sufficiently improved to be regarded as 'remitted' or 'recovered'.

Internalising personality   A style of dealing with stress by not discussing things openly. Instead, individuals with this personality style become quiet, go to their room, cry quietly and exhibit other withdrawal behaviours.

Maintenance therapy   Usually a term restricted to drug therapies that are either in place, or are put into place, after a patient's episode has been brought under control. Such therapies are designed to prevent the onset of any new episode.

Major depression   A DSM diagnosis describing an episode of depression with a certain number of specific features present for two weeks or more and associated with social impairment.

Mania   A high mood that is of distinct severity and where the individual is commonly psychotic (that is, with delusions and/or hallucinations).

Melancholia   The quintessential 'biological' depressive sub-type, it has been variously described as: likely to emerge without any antecedent stressor; having certain clinical features (such as observable PMD) and having over-represented features (for example, non-reactive mood, anhedonia, mood worse in the morning); having genetic determinants; providing strong evidence of biological determinants; being unlikely to respond to placebo medication; and being highly likely to respond to physical treatments.

Minor depression   A DSM category for disorders not severe enough to meet the criteria for major depression. Including dysthymia as well as several brief depressive disorders.

Mixed states   A term used to describe those with bipolar disorder who may have features of both mania and depression at the same time or who switch from one of those states to the other.

Mood   Either a personal description of how the individual feels (contrasting with affect or how the individual appears), or a reference to a more persistent emotional state than an affect.

Mood stabilisers   These are drugs that help control the fluctuations of mood that typify bipolar disorder.

Neuroleptic   A drug used in the treatment of any disorders with psychotic phenomena.

Neurotic depression   A dated term used to describe a depressive sub-type contrasted with endogenous depression. It referred to individuals with personality styles (for example, neurotic, highly anxious, shy and unassertive) that disposed them to a greater risk of depression when faced with a life event stressor.

Neurotransmitters   Chemical substances present in the brain that help carry signals between nerve cells. These can become depleted, or otherwise get out of balance, and so lead to mental disorders.

Noradrenaline   A catecholamine neurotransmitter.

Pharmacotherapy   Drug therapy.

Physical treatment   This is a term for treatments that have physical concomitants (for example, drug or ECT treatment) as opposed to psychological interventions.

Post-natal depression   Any type of depression in the first nine to twelve months following the birth of a baby.

Post-partum blues   A mild post-natal depression generally occurring in the first few weeks after having a baby.

Post-partum or **puerperal psychosis**   Any psychotic condition occurring in the first few weeks after having a baby, and most commonly a depressive (or manic) disorder rather than a schizophrenic disorder.

Primary and secondary conditions   The term primary (as in 'primary depression') indicates that this condition provides the first, major or largest input to the presenting problems. Secondary depression generally indicates that the depression follows, or is otherwise related to, another major medical condition, be it psychiatric (for example, schizophrenia), medical (for example, a stroke) or other (for example, alcohol state).

Proximal stressor   A stressful situation occurring immediately prior to a depressive episode that may have caused its onset.

Psychomotor disturbance   Decreased movement (that is, retardation) or increased or perturbed movement (that is, agitation) observable in melancholic and psychotic depression, but absent in non-melancholic depression.

Psychopharmacology   The science relating to drug therapy for psychiatric disorders.

Psychosis   An impairment of mental functioning in which the individual loses touch with reality and usually experiences delusions and/or hallucinations.

Psychotherapy   A non-physical treatment whereby the therapist adopts a particular structure (for example, analytic, interpersonal, cognitive, cognitive-behavioural) to address symptoms and/or personality problems experienced by an individual. It has a number of non-specific components (for example, empathy) that may be therapeutic in themselves.

Psychotic depression   Either a sub-class of melancholic depression or a separate sub-type altogether. Clinical features involve those most commonly over-represented in melancholic depression, including observable PMD, although these features are generally more severe, with the added presence of psychotic symptoms (that is, delusions and/or hallucinations).

Reactive depression   An old term to describe those whose depressive episode appears entirely explainable as a consequence of having experienced a major stress, and with the implication that its clinical pattern is not melancholic in type. Now less popular, as life event stress has been found to have minimal specificity to any depressive sub-type.

Recovery   When an individual's depressive episode has completely resolved for a defined period.

Recurrence   When an individual has been completely well from depression for a defined period and then develops a new episode.

Relapse   When an individual has not completely recovered from an earlier episode of depression and there is the return of a full episode.

Remission   When an individual's episode of depression (or mania) has resolved completely but the period has been so brief that it is not clear whether or not the actual 'recovery' has occurred.

Schizo-affective disorder   A term used to describe a clinical pattern combining some features of schizophrenia in conjunction with those of a mood disorder (either mania or depression), and most commonly used when the exact diagnosis remains unclear.

Schizophrenia   A psychiatric condition where delusions and hallucinations are common; thinking, insight and attention commonly impaired; with behavioural problems frequent. A condition quite distinct from the mood disorders, although a significant percentage of those with schizophrenia develop a superimposed depression.

Seasonal affective disorder   A pattern where depressive episodes occur on a reasonably regular basis in particular seasons (especially autumn and winter) and remit in the alternate seasons (spring and summer). The clinical feature pattern may differ from classic depression (for example, by hypersomnia or appetite increase). Phototherapy ('bright light' therapy) may be effective. This condition is more common in the northern hemisphere, but it does exist in Australia.

Secondary depression   Where the depression follows some physical condition (for example, a stroke) or substance abuse; or in some cases is a by-product of or co-existent with some other psychiatric condition (such as schizophrenia).

Serotonin   A neurotransmitter (otherwise known as 5-HT or 5-Hydroxytryptamine) that is widely distributed in the body, as well as in the brain.

Side-effects   Some unintended effects of medication that can exist alongside the positive effects of the drug. These are more discernable in the older style antidepressants than the newer medications. If side-effects are too disruptive, then medication dosages may have to be lowered or that medication ceased. Side-effects are usually most pronounced in the first few weeks of treatment, but then settle down after that.

Somatic   To do with the body, for example, a physical illness.

Spontaneous remission   When an individual's episode of depression (or mania) has seemingly resolved completely and without medical intervention.

Stigma   The experience of depression can be painful because of a sense of shame felt as people attempt to fulfil their accustomed roles in the face of discrimination practised by the wider community. There are programs aimed at destigmatising depression so that people can feel positive about seeking help.

Stressor   An event or interpersonal interaction that causes distress to an individual. Stressors can be acute (for example, the immediate aftermath of an accident) or chronic (for example, poverty, a poor marriage).

Stupor   A state of reduced consciousness.

Unipolar depression   Originally used to sub-classify the behaviour pattern of those with melancholic depression who have only had depressive episodes over time (in contrast to those with bipolar depression). The term is now used essentially to describe the longitudinal course of any 'non-bipolar' condition.

Vegetative features   Certain symptoms (for example, appetite and weight loss) that are more somatic than psychological and that are commonly reported by those with depressive disorders.

References and further resources

Refer to Mood Disorders Unit and Black Dog institute Website, *http://www.mdu.unsw.edu.au* for further references.

☆ Medication

Relevant information can be obtained from medical encyclopaedias, or by access to bimonthly and annual MIMS (*http://www.mims.com.au*), or to an internet drug index that provides non-technical information on more than 4500 drugs in common usage (*http://www.RxList.com*).

☆ Australian Websites of interest

Depression

http://www.mdu.unsw.edu.au
This Website for the Mood Disorders Unit provides a range of further references not listed here.
http://www.healthinsite.gov.au
This site provides a listing of Australian-only health sites that have been assessed as credible by the Department of Health and Aged Care.
http://www.beyondblue.org.au
The site for the 'beyond blue' national depression initiative.

http://mentalhealth.anu.edu.au
Developed by the Centre for Mental Health Research (ANU, Canberra) and the CSIRO Division of Mathematical and Information Sciences, this Website is designed to provide information about depression.

http://moodgym.anu.edu.au
Developed by the Centre for Mental Health Research (ANU, Canberra), this Website provides an Internet-based CBT intervention.

http://depressioNet.com.au
DepressioNet aims to be a one-stop depression information resource for Australians. The site also includes information about new research and opportunities to contribute to this research.

Bipolar disorder

http://www.nswamh.org/dmda
This is the Website of the Depression and Mood Disorders Association of NSW. Its objective is to inform and help people with bipolar disorder, depression or mood disorders, their families and friends.

http://members.iinet.net.au/~fractal1/fhello.htm
Fyreniyce refers to itself as 'The Australian Bipolar Website', a site dedicated to those who suffer from bipolar disorder. The goal is to learn about the disorder, develop constructive ways to deal with it and provide support for those affected.

General

http://www.sane.org
This Website is run by SANE, an Australian charity helping people affected by mental illness, through lobbying, education and research. It offers an information and referral service.

http://healthnetwork.com.au
The Health Network is an Australian and New Zealand resource centre. Its health information database is separated into life stages but also allows browsing by condition and treatment.

http://www.health.gov.au
This is the Website of the Australian Department of Health and Aged

Care. It has information on policy initiatives, current campaigns and publications.

☆ USA Websites of interest

Depression

http://www.psycom.net/depression.central.html
Dr Ivan's Depression Central, as this site is called, aims to operate as a 'clearinghouse' for information about major depression, manic depression (bipolar disorder), cyclothymia, dysthymia and other mood disorders and their effective treatment.
http://www.human-nature.com/odmh/depression.html
This is the online Dictionary of Mental Health. It also provides links to other sites that enlarge on topics discussed.
http://www.sciam.com/1998/0698issue/0698nemeroff.html
This site for *Scientific American* carries a comprehensive article on the neurobiology of depression.
http://www.depression.org
National Foundation for Depressive Illness Inc. (NAFDI) provides information about depression, referral and support groups.
http://www.nami.org
National Alliance for the Mentally Ill (NAMI) provides support, information and referral.
http://www.mgh.harvard.edu or
http://www.healthcare.partners.org/depression
The Depression Clinical and Research Program at the Massachusetts General Hospital provides information on depression and how to become involved in research studies.

Bipolar disorder

http://www/med.jhu.edu/drada/creativity.html
DRADA (Depression and Related Affective Disorders Association) provides education, information and support to those with depression and bipolar illness, including support groups, training, book reviews and research articles.
http://www.mgh.harvard.edu or
http://www.massgeneral.org/allpsych/bipolar/index.html

The Harvard Bipolar Program offers information on living with bipolar disorder, care providers and getting involved in research.
http://www.ndmda.org
The National Depressive and Manic Depressive Association aims to inform that all depressive and manic-depressive illness are treatable medical diseases, as well as to foster self-help, improve access to care, and advocate for research to eliminate these illnesses.

General

http://healthfinder.gov
'Healthfinder'®is a service of the US Department of Health and Human Services. It aims to be a provider of reliable health information.
http://mayohealth.org
This Website, connected with the Mayo Clinic, provides information about general diseases and advice on taking charge of your own health, plus news items of health interest and answers to questions put to specialists.
http://www.onhealth.com
This Website describes itself as a 'new way to look at everything' and covers everything from diseases to alternative health and lifestyle advice for women, family and babies.
http://www.nmha.org
National Mental Health Association (NMHA) addresses all aspects of mental health and mental illness through advocacy, education, research and service.

☆ Canadian Websites of interest

http://www.fhs.mcmaster.ca/direct
Depression and Anxiety Information Resource and Education.
http://www.depressioncanada.com
This Website provides information on symptoms of depression, treatment and medications.
http://www.mentalhealth.com/dis/p20-md01.html
This site aims to improve understanding, diagnosis and treatment of mental illness, and to provide information about effective, well-researched treatments.

http://www.mentalhealth.com/dis/p20-md02.html
This site aims to provide information about diagnosis, characteristics
and treatment of bipolar disorder.

☆ UK Websites of interest

*http://www.psychiatry.ox.ac.uk/cebmh/guidelines/depression/depress
ion1.html*
A systematic guide for the management of depression in primary care
from the Centre for Evidence-Based Mental Health (Oxford).
http://cebmh.warne.ox.ac.uk/cebmh/ebmh/depression or
http://www.nhsdirect.nhs.uk/depression
This National Health Service facility provides information on depression and support organisations.
http://www.depressionalliance.org
This Website contains useful information about different types of
depression, medical treatment, and self help.

☆ Accessing other Websites

There are numerous websites providing information on depression
and mental health. They can be accessed via search engines, by
entering search terms such as 'depression' or 'mental health', and if
required for a particular country, by including the name (or abbre-
viation) of that country in the search term (e.g. uk depression). For
more specific searches related to depression, include the topic of
interest in the search term (e.g. uk depression treatment; uk depression medications; uk depression symptoms; uk depression self-help).

☆ Key references

Mood Disorders Unit publications

Austin, M.P. 'Psychotropic medications in pregnant women: update and treatment guidelines', *Medical Journal of Australia*, 169, pp. 428–31, 1998.

Loo, C., Mitchell, P., Sachdev, P., McDarmont, B., Parker, G. and Gandevia, S. 'Double-blind controlled investigation of transcranial magnetic stimulation for the treatment of resistant major depression', *American Journal of Psychiatry*, 156, 6, pp. 946–8.

Mitchell, P. 'The use of psychotropic medications in breast-feeding women: acute and prophylactic treatment', *Australian and New Zealand Journal of Psychiatry*, 32, pp. 778–84, 1998.

—— 'Managing depression in a community setting', *Medical Journal of Australia*, 167, pp. 383–8.

Parker G. 'Can paradigms lost be regained?' *American Journal of Psychiatry* 157, pp. 1204–11, 2000.

Parker G. and Hadzi-Pavlovic D. (eds) *Melancholia: A Disorder of Movement and Mood*, Cambridge University Press, New York, 1996.

Parker, G., Hadzi-Pavlovic, D., Roussos, J., Wilhelm, K., Mitchell, P., Austen, M-P., Hickie, I., Gladstone, G. and Eyers, K. 'Non-melancholic depression: the contribution of personality, anxiety and life events to subclassification', *Psychological Medicine*, 28, pp. 1209–19.

Wilhelm, K. 'Depression 2000: an update for general practitioners', *Australian Doctor*, 4 February.

Other publications

Abrams, R. *Electroconvulsive Therapy*, 2nd edn, Oxford University Press, Oxford, 1992.

Bethlehem and Maudsley Trust *The Maudsley Prescribing Guidelines*, 5th edn, Martin Dunitz, London, 1999.

George, M.S. & Bellmaker, R.M. *Transcranial Magnetic Stimulation in Psychiatry*, American Psychiatric Association Press, Inc., Washington, 2000.

Jamison, K. *Touched with Fire: Manic-Depressive Illness and the Artistic Temperament*, The Free Press, New York, 1993.

—— *An Unquiet Mind: A Memoir of Moods and Madness*, Alfred A. Knopf Inc., New York, 1995.

—— *Night Falls Fast: Understanding Suicide*, Alfred A. Knopf Inc., New York, 1999.

Milligan, S. and Clare, A. *Depression and How to Survive It*, Arrow Books, London, 1994.

MIMS Manuals, Medimedia Australia Pty Ltd, St Leonards, Sydney.

Nesse, R.M. 'Is depression an adaptation?' *Archives of General Psychiatry*, 57, pp. 14–20.

Orum, M. 'Van Gogh and lithium. Creativity and bipolar disorder: perspective of a psychologist/writer', *Australian and New Zealand Journal of Psychiatry*, vol. 33 (supplement) S114–S116, 1999.

Razor, H. *Gas Smells Awful: The Mechanics of Being a Nutcase*, Random House, Sydney, 1999.

Rowe, P. 'Van Gogh and lithium. Creativity and bipolar disorder: perspective of a writer', *Australian and New Zealand Journal of Psychiatry*, vol. 33 (supplement) S117–S119, 1999.

Styron, W. *Darkness Visible*, Picador, London, 1992.

Tanner, S. and Ball, J. *Beating the Blues: A Self-help Approach to Overcoming Depression*, Tower Books, Sydney, 1999.

Victorian Medical Postgraduate Foundation Therapeutic Committee *Psychotropic Drug Guidelines*, 3rd edn, 1996.

Weissman, M.M. *Patient's Handbook for Depression*, Harcourt Brace, Sydney, 1995.

Williams, J. et al. *Annals of Internal Medicine*, vol. 132, pp. 743–56.

Wolpert, L. *Malignant Sadness: The Anatomy of Depression*, Faber & Faber Ltd, London, 1999.

Index

psychotic phenomena *see* delusions; hallucinations
Psychotropic Drug Guidelines 85
puerperal psychosis 37, 40–1, 132

rational thinking 94–6
Razor, Helen 35, 36, 105
recklessness 32, 47, 49
recurrence, of depression 121, 133
relapse 133
relationship breakdown 17, 43–4, 57
reliability 48
resentment 109, 119
resilience 47, 103
responsibility 48
  irrational 94
retardation 7, 33–4, 35, 35–6, 64
risk factors
  distal 54–6
  proximal 56–9
Rowe, Penelope 122

St John's Wort 78–9
schemas 91–2
schizophrenia 40, 133
seasonal affective disorder 56, 133–4
selective serotonin reuptake inhibitors (SSRIs) 75, 76–7, 114
self-confidence 37, 51
self-esteem 6, 33, 41, 44, 48, 51, 55, 57, 68
self-talk 53, 96
self-worth 57, 102
sensitivity, interpersonal 49–50
separation anxiety 42, 43
serotonin 50, 65, 66, 67–8, 75, 134
serotonin-dopamine antagonists (SDAs) 80–1
sex drive 7, 8, 37
shyness 48, 50, 69
side-effects
  of drugs 85, 134
  of ECT 88
sleep disturbance 6, 8, 20, 42, 43–4, 66
  excessive sleep 13, 50, 130
smell, sense of 7, 36
social class 55

social engineering 69
social interaction 48, 98
social phobia 42, 51
speech patterns 34, 36, 37
spontaneous remission 20, 22, 134
  in melancholic depression 115
  in non-melancholic depression 112
  in psychotic melancholia 116
stigma 9, 61, 123, 134
stress 54, 56, 59, 109
  and counselling 104
  and melancholic depression 58–9
  and non-melancholic depression 22, 56, 57
  and psychotic melancholia 58–9
stressors 58–9, 134
  distal 54–6, 128
  proximal 56–9, 132
Styron, William 34, 35, 122
sub-typing 10, 16–18, 64, 66, 67, 118
substance abuse 56, 121
Sudden Infant Death Syndrome (SIDS) 44
suicide 33, 36, 41, 49, 66, 121–2
  thoughts of 7, 32, 120
symptom formation 98
synapses 65, 66, 67–8

Tanner, Susan 97
task-orientation 47
taste, sense of 7, 36
temperament
  defined 46
  dimensions 47
The Maudsley Prescribing Guidelines 85
therapeutic relationship 103
thinking habits 91
  faulty 93–4
    arbitrary inference 94
    black and white thinking 93
    generalising 93
    losing sense of proportion 93–4
    personalising 94
    selective abstraction 94
    unrealistic expectations 94
  irrational beliefs 95–6
  positive thinking 94–5